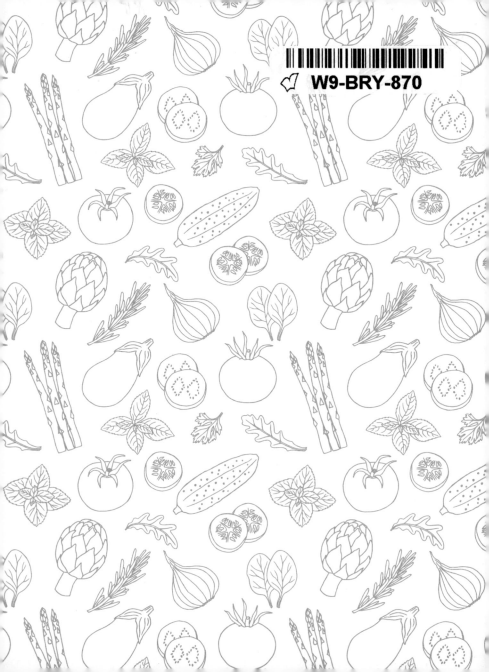

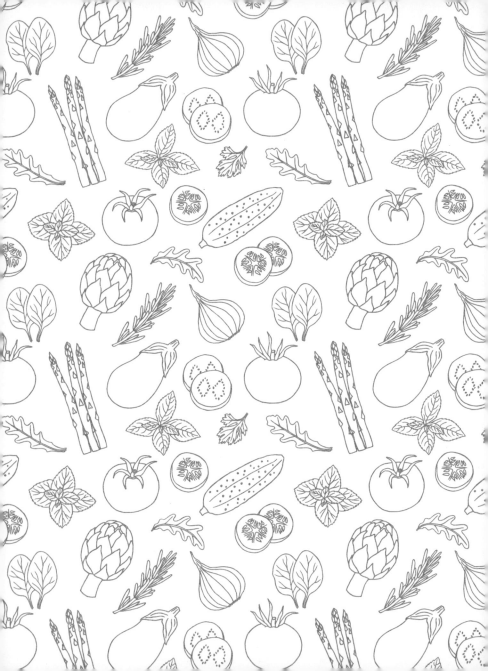

THIS JOURNAL BELONGS TO:

_____

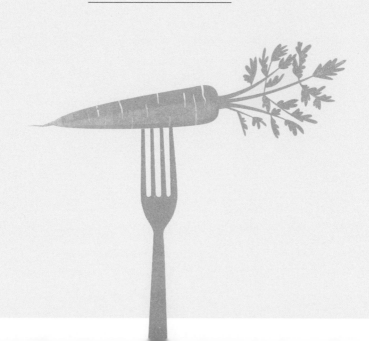

THE
skinnytaste™
MEAL PLANNER

POTTER STYLE
NEW YORK

About This Journal

When I started trying to lose weight a few years ago, I found that the two things that made the biggest difference were cooking fresh, from-scratch, healthy dinners at home, where I was in control of what went into my meals, and tracking everything I ate so I knew exactly what (and how much) I was eating. Cooking greatly improved the quality and taste of my meals, and tracking helped clue me in to what foods to eat, what foods to limit, and how to make healthier daily choices.

So many readers of my blog Skinnytaste.com and my cookbook, *The Skinnytaste Cookbook*, are smart, proactive people who are ready to make a change in the name of health. That's why they like my recipes, which are not only full-flavored, but also surprisingly low in fat and calories—so you don't feel like you're eating diet food or missing out on the good stuff. After all, if you don't enjoy the process, it isn't likely to become a lifelong habit! With these types of folks in mind, I've created *The Skinnytaste Meal Planner*.

This journal is a daily tool to help you plan your meals and track your eating, as well as schedule your exercise activities, throughout the week. In the Weekly Meal Planner pages, you have a bird's-eye view of the week; this is where you can decide what days you have time to cook, which days will be leftover dinners, and how to otherwise organize your approach to cooking for the week.

On the Caloric/Points Tracker pages, there's space to write down all the foods you eat each day, along with a place to log the amount of calories or points consumed. That way, you can see just how much is coming in—and you'll see if one particular meal or snack is throwing you off your goal! The last page of each week includes a box for tracking your exercise, since being active and burning calories day by day is also essential to being healthy.

Throughout the journal I've included motivational quotes, which get me going on days when I really need it. An inspirational phrase can instantly fill me with optimism and help me make good on my promises to myself! There are also notes on everyday superfoods—certain ingredients that are nutritional powerhouses—as well as twenty recipes, each using one of these important foods, so you can work them into your eating.

Taking charge of your cooking and eating habits can make a big impact on your health and weight. I hope that *The Skinnytaste Meal Planner* is a helpful tool for you to get on the road to your very best self—and have fun while you're at it!

HOW TO USE THIS PLANNER AND TRACKER

I truly believe that the best way to achieve your goals is to hold yourself accountable along the way. And diet and exercise are no exception! When I began my journey years ago, I was shocked by what I learned when I actually wrote down what I ate in a day. I'd always thought I ate lean and light, and that I was fairly active. But I realized that every day I was inadvertently sneaking in bites of food that added up fast, and that my "exercise" didn't actually burn any calories of note. Seeing the real deal on paper made me snap to it! I finally knew where I was slipping up and why I wasn't seeing results—then I was able to determine how to get things under control.

The two sections of this journal are meant to work in tandem.

Meal Planner

At the beginning of the week, state what your goal (or goals) for that week is (are)—what do you want to try to do, more or less, during that week? Do you want to try a new food, or go cold turkey on sugar-packed sodas? Maybe you want to try swapping in almond milk for full-fat cow's milk, or be more diligent in packing healthy snacks to take to work so that you don't visit the vending machine every afternoon. Be creative in this section and think of things that challenge you to be mindful whenever you eat. And you can even write exercise goals here, too! Do you want to try a spin class for the first time, or walk with a friend three mornings a week? Write it down. At the end of the week, you can review your goals and see if you followed through—or decide if you should carry a goal into the next week.

Next, plan your meals for the week with your goal or goals in mind. No matter how much any of us loves to cook, it still takes a good amount of planning and preparing to pull off! With busy schedules and the rigors of grocery shopping, being proactive will help you succeed. When I was losing weight, I found that I ate healthier foods when I was in control of the dishes—and that meant cooking. Aim for a certain number of days to cook each week, and write out which days those will be. Then you'll be better able to arrange other things in your week so that you also have time to cook. Also, come up with some ideas for your leftovers! I love it when I make a little extra of a dish so that I can enjoy it again later in the week—either just as they are, or remade into another delicious dish. Leftovers are great to pack for work, too. Another way to use the planner is to map out your snacks. It can be easy to fall into a rut of having one thing everyday—or turning to the vending machine or nabbing your kids' snacks!—so giving a little thought to snacks beforehand will set you on the right road.

Calorie/Points and Exercise Tracker

After planning, it's time to be accountable! And that's where the tracker pages come in the picture. As I said before, it's one thing to think you eat healthfully, but it's another thing to know for sure. Use these pages to write down every single thing you eat in a day. Did you skip breakfast? Okay, but don't do that again (breakfast is important!). A colleague brought in cookies and you had half of one? Write it down! You'll be surprised to see how many little things like these accumulate. You'll notice that there are spaces grouped under the letters B, L, D, and S. Those stand for Breakfast, Lunch, Dinner, and Snacks. In the space next to where you wrote down each dish or item of food consumed, add the calories of those foods. This is where your eyes may be opened! Sometimes a seemingly innocent sandwich from your local shop is a calorie bomb in disguise. And sometimes you'll find that your salad is healthier than you thought! It'll probably go both ways, and by tracking these calorie counts, you'll begin to find a way to better tailor your eating so that you stay fit and only indulge in comfort foods every now and again.

Don't forget to exercise! Moving your body is just as pivotal to overall health as eating well is, so don't neglect this side of the equation. Aim for at least 20 minutes of exercise most days of the week—and work your way up to more! Have fun with it. Join a running group so your exercise time is social, or find a fun class at your gym to keep you motivated. Craft a new playlist to keep your energy high, and get a couple of new tank tops (hey, looking good can help you feel good!). There are so many ways to accumulate data on how many calories you burned by performing various activities, from the counters on gym machines to those handy personal trackers like FitBit. You can also go online to MyFitnessPal.com/exercise/lookup for information on calories burned that takes into account your weight.

Above all, I hope that this journal is helpful to you. Feeling confident in yourself, being active and fit, and knowing that you're fueling your body with the best foods possible will boost your happiness. And accomplishing your goals will give you a surge of joy that will spread throughout your life! Check out my examples of how to fill in this journal on the pages that follow the "11 Easy Ways" section.

Getting Started

It can be difficult to take those first steps toward a healthier lifestyle—I've been there and know firsthand! But all you need to do is start simple: learn what foods are truly good for you and how many calories you need per day, and then work in changes to your eating and exercise week by week.

So, how do you know how many calories you're supposed to aim for each day? This is a good first question to answer, since that number will be your main guide to shedding weight. If you're following a points-based plan, then you know how important calories are, and you're likely familiar with how many you should be consuming. A basic rule of thumb is that an average adult woman should consume 1,500 to 1,600 calories per day in order to see a healthy weight loss of approximately two pounds per week. Bear in mind, though, that many factors, such as height, weight, and activity level, greatly influence this number. There are great calorie calculators online; I recommend checking out www.mayoclinic.org/calorie-calculator/itt-20084939 to find the right daily caloric intake for you.

11 EASY WAYS TO EAT CLEAN

Health before weight loss is my first priority, so eating clean is always my main focus. And by cleaning your diet and focusing on foods that make your calories count, the pounds will naturally come off. Work on eating the healthiest options in each food group (fresh fruits and vegetables, lean protein, good fats, and whole grains) while eliminating from your diet the not-so-healthy ones (processed foods, refined grains, refined sugars, and unhealthy fats). Here are a few simple tips to get you started and reprogram your eating habits.

1. Read Your Labels

The first step to cleaning up your diet is to limit or avoid the amount of processed or refined foods you consume. This is easier than you think. Look at the ingredient list on the back of the packaged foods before you purchase them. If there's a long list of ingredients (more than five), or if there are ingredients you can't pronounce, stay away. If you're unsure the next time you're in the supermarket, I highly recommend the smart phone app called Fooducate, which lets you scan the items in the supermarket, and then the app grades the food, explains the ingredients listed, and suggests healthier alternatives.

2. Homemade Is Healthier

Although it takes a little more time, cooking your favorite foods—such as macaroni and cheese, marinara sauce, bread crumbs, granola bars, and baked goods—rather than buying them from a box or the frozen aisle will not only be cleaner and healthier, they'll taste better, too. Again, check the label to see how many unnatural foods are hiding in that frozen apple pie!

3. Drink More Water

Our bodies need water for everything! Drinking enough water is key to feeling great. And did you know that sometimes thirst can be mistaken for hunger? Make sure you don't reach for a snack when what you really need is a glass of water! Your goal should be to drink approximately 2 liters a day. If you're in the habit of drinking soda, try switching to seltzer that you flavor with fresh-squeezed citrus or fresh mint.

4. Eat More Veggies
On average, as a nation, we are still behind the daily recommended intake of vegetables, which is 2½ to 3 cups for adults. Make it a goal to increase your veggie consumption, and you'll be adding healthful vitamins, minerals, and fiber every day. And try going meatless once a week! Meatless Mondays are a great way to focus on veggie meals and can make it fun for your family, too.

5. Choose Organic When Possible
Nowadays, organic fruits and vegetables are widely available. Most grocery stores, and even Walmart, stock lots of clean produce. The more organic foods you eat, the less you fill your body with harmful chemicals. If it's not in your budget to eat everything organic, at least try to avoid the Environmental Working Group's Dirty Dozen: apples, celery, cherry tomatoes, cucumbers, grapes, nectarines, peaches, potatoes, snap peas, spinach, strawberries, and sweet bell peppers.

6. Choose Lean Protein
Nothing will keep you feeling full like protein! It's necessary for muscle growth, too, and is a must every day. Focus on eating lean proteins so that you keep calories low while getting the good stuff. Lean proteins include: chicken breast, eggs, legumes, tofu, edamame, turkey, roast beef, pork tenderloin, Greek yogurt, low-fat milk, cottage cheese, nuts and nut butters, seeds, and fish.

7. Opt for Whole Grains
We are so lucky these days that grocery stores stock a wide variety of excellent whole grains, which are leaps and bounds more healthy than their processed counterparts. Reach for oatmeal and brown rice, whole wheat bread, granola, quinoa, barley, farro, bulgur, spelt, and more.

8. Snack on More Fruit

So many foods advertised today as "snacks" have us reaching for crackers, chips, cookies, and other carbs—many of which are loaded with salt and refined sugars. Reach instead for fresh fruits, which have natural sugars, as well as lots of vitamins, minerals, and fiber. Pack them in your bag so that you're always armed when hunger strikes!

9. Consume Healthy Fats

Not all fat is bad for you! That's a myth of the past, but now we know that many healthy fats are excellent parts of a good diet. Some foods with good fats to work into your weekly eating are olives, salmon, avocados, nuts, nut butter, pumpkin seeds, sesame seeds, and olive oil.

10. Cut Back on Sugar

It is amazing the things that are packed with sugar these days! Sugar is almost a way of life for Americans, but thankfully the word is out that too much in your diet can harm your health in many ways—and lots of people are learning to make better choices. Aim to decrease the sugar you consume a little every day. A great place to start is by eliminating soda. You'll avoid about 44 grams of sugar per can of cola!

11. Limit Your Cocktails

I love a good cocktail or glass of wine at the end of the day, and especially when out with girlfriends! But I also know that drinks can be extremely high in calories—more than 200 calories for one drink! Even a glass of red wine has about 125. The caloric impact of cocktails adds up fast, so aim to limit your consumption and avoid sugary drinks.

Weekly Meal Planner

Weekly Goals _____

Workout 4 days

Drink more water

Try a new gym class!

MON

Grilled Lamb Chops with Mint Yogurt Sauce
Quinoa Tabbouleh

TUE

Skinny Broccoli Mac and Cheese
House Salad Made with Love

WED

Coconut Chicken Salad
Piña Colada Chia Pudding

THU

Skinny Chicken Parmesan
Lemon Roasted Asparagus

FRI

Pizza night! Order from Nick's

SAT

So-Addicted Chicken Enchiladas

SUN

Chocolate Chip Pancakes
Slow Cooker Picadillo

Calories/Points Tracker

DAILY GOAL **1,600**

FOODS	CALORIES/POINTS
B Coffee with	
1 tsp sugar	18
1 oz milk	18
2 eggs	166
1 ww toast	80
Banana	105
L Greek salad	300
3 oz grilled	
chicken	154

FOODS	CALORIES/POINTS
D Lamb chops	248
Quinoa tabbouleh	154
S 1 oz cheddar	114
1 oz cashews	162
Peach	59
TOTAL CALORIES/POINTS	**1,534**

MON

FOODS	CALORIES/POINTS
B Coffee with	
1 tsp sugar	18
1 oz milk	18
Green Monster	
smoothie	254
L Leftover quinoa	
tabbouleh	110
Pita	160
Apple	91

FOODS	CALORIES/POINTS
D Broccoli mac	
and cheese	321
House salad	117
S 1 cup cherries	87
1 oz pistachios	160
1 oz chocolate	149
1 tbsp peanut	96
butter	
TOTAL CALORIES/POINTS	**1,572**

TUE

DATE **5 / 11 / 15** TO **5 / 17 / 15**

WED

FOODS	CALORIES/POINTS
8 oz 0% Greek	
B yogurt	130
1 tbsp honey	64
½ oz walnuts	93
Coffee with	
1 tsp sugar	18
1 oz milk	18
L Egg, tomato,	
scallion	
sandwich	220

FOODS	CALORIES/POINTS
D Coconut chicken	
salad	340
6 oz white wine	142
S Piña colada	
chia pudding	161
Banana	105
Chai tea latte	240
TOTAL CALORIES/POINTS	**1,592**

THU

FOODS	CALORIES/POINTS
B PB&J overnight	
oats	288
2 coffees with	
2 tsp sugar	32
2 oz milk	32
L 2 oz ww bread	
w/ 2 oz canned	
tuna, ¼ avocado,	
tomato, and	
sprouts	300
Peach	59

FOODS	CALORIES/POINTS
D Chicken	
parmesan	174
2 oz pasta	200
Lemon asparagus	
(2 servings)	48
6 oz white wine	142
S Banana	105
5 oz yogurt	87
1 tbsp jam	10
TOTAL CALORIES/POINTS	**1,538**

HEALTHY AND DELICIOUS INGREDIENTS SWAPS

One of my best Skinnytaste tricks is to swap out full-fat ingredients or those with empty calories for more nutritious items. You still get amazing flavor, with the bonus of better-for-you food! Here's a list of my favorite swaps to help you learn how to take your favorite recipes from diet saboteur to skinny.

↪ **SWAP** Mashed avocado *for* mayo

Move over, mayo. Not only does avocado deliver monounsaturated fat, which helps protect the heart, and vitamin E, which is vital to immune function, but it also has nearly half the calories and fat of mayo. A 2-tablespoon serving of mayo has around 200 calories and 20 grams of fat, while that of a mashed avocado has only around 120 calories and 10 grams of fat.

↪ **SWAP** Greek yogurt *for* mayo

Save calories and fat without sacrificing flavor. Greek yogurt has the same creamy consistency of mayo, but it offers some protein, which is more satiating than fat and carbs. Add a bit of red wine vinegar, and use it in place of mayo in mayonnaise-based salads. Or make a more conservative change: Swap out half the mayo for yogurt—you won't notice the difference.

↪ **SWAP** Egg whites *for* whole eggs

When I make a dish that requires eggs, such as egg salad or omelets, I replace half of the whole eggs with egg whites. This allows me to cut back on cholesterol while still getting a healthy helping of satiating protein. I don't go totally yolk-free though, because there are some healthful nutrients (like the antioxidants lutein and zeaxanthin and the B vitamin choline) in the yolk.

↪ **SWAP** Lettuce leaves *for* wraps or tortillas

Using fresh lettuce in place of wraps or tortillas is an easy way to cut your carb intake and increase the nutrition value of your meal. My favorite lettuce to use for this purpose is iceberg lettuce because the outer leaves are large and the texture is crisp. You can also try using Romaine, Boston, or even cabbage.

↻ SWAP Mashed cauliflower *for* mashed potatoes

Steamed and mashed cauliflower has a very similar texture to mashed potatoes. But cauliflower is, well, a head above the potato because it's lower in calories and it may help protect against heart disease and cancer.

↻ SWAP Zucchini "noodles" *for* pasta

I use a spiralizer or a mandolin fitted with a julienne blade to cut zucchini into spaghetti-like strands. You can also use a potato peeler to cut them into ribbons (just make sure you leave out the "seedy" part in the middle or they end up too mushy). You can eat the strands raw, but I like to season them with salt and pepper and sauté them in a little oil for about 2 minutes. A good rule of thumb is to make one medium 8-ounce zucchini per person because it shrinks a little when it cooks.

↻ SWAP Spaghetti squash *for* pasta

Talk about a calorie savings: One cup of pasta has 220 calories, whereas a cup of spaghetti squash has only 42 calories. Plus, that cup of spaghetti squash is much more nutrient-dense, meaning it contains a lot more vitamins and minerals. Roast or microwave the squash, and then use a fork to pull apart and separate the spaghetti-like strands. The result: a slimmer, healthier alternative to pasta in the fall and winter months.

↻ SWAP Ground turkey or chicken *for* ground beef

There are times when I still prefer to cook with lean ground beef, but most of the time I replace the beef with ground turkey or chicken to cut back on saturated fat. It works for meat loaf, meatballs, chili, burgers, and more.

↻ SWAP Brown rice *for* white rice

To produce white rice (which keeps longer than brown rice), manu-facturers strip the kernel of its outer layer, also known as the bran. Unfortunately, that's where you'll find many of the good-for-you nutrients, including fiber and B vitamins. Stick with brown rice for the extra fiber and vitamins. Dried brown rice takes a little longer to cook than white; if you're short on time, buy parboiled brown rice, which is ready in about 10 minutes.

↻ SWAP Whole-grain bread *for* white bread

Replacing processed white bread with whole-grain bread is a simple way to get more vitamins, fiber, and vital nutrients. Although food producers try to add these health-promoting nutrients back to the product after processing, these unnatural sources are not as easily absorbed and digested by the body.

↻ SWAP Whole-grain pasta *for* white pasta

Whole-grain pasta has come a long way over the years. I find the flavor to be richer than white pasta, and it's certainly healthier—you'll get more fiber and vitamins by opting for whole grain. Nowadays, there are more choices than ever, including whole wheat pasta, brown rice pasta, and quinoa pasta, to name just a few.

↻ SWAP Oil mister *for* oil direct from a bottle

Oil helps add flavor and keeps food from sticking during the cooking process, but it's loaded with fat and calories. What's a chef to do? Try misting instead of pouring. I use at least three oil misters—one for olive oil, one for canola oil, and one for sesame oil. Remember, a little goes a long way.

↻ SWAP Oven frying *for* deep frying

You can achieve the same crispy golden texture you get from frying right in your own oven. It's easier, quicker, and (bonus!) there's no greasy mess to clean up.

↻ SWAP Avocado puree *for* butter

Avocado, which is creamy and nearly flavorless, can be used as a healthier stand-in for butter in cookies, cakes, and brownies. Avocados are loaded with vitamin E and heart-protecting monounsaturated fat, so you can feel a little less guilty about enjoying your splurge. You can generally swap equal amounts of well-mashed avocado for butter.

↻ SWAP Unsweetened applesauce *for* oil or butter

Applesauce is another great substitution for butter when making muffins, quick breads, and even pancakes. Plus, it adds some natural sweetness, so you can cut back on the sugar. **NOTE:** *Because applesauce doesn't contain fat, you still have to keep some of the butter or oil. It takes some experimenting to figure out how much to cut out. If you're making a favorite indulgent*

recipe, try swapping half the fat for
applesauce the first time you make
it, and then adjust accordingly the
next time.

⟲ SWAP Ripe mashed bananas *for* oil or butter

Like avocados and applesauce, bananas have a creamy consistency that makes them an ideal replacement for fats in muffins, quick breads, and pancakes. They also add moisture and sweetness, so you can use less sugar. Another benefit: You'll get some potassium, fiber, and a handful of vitamins. Start by replacing half the fat with mashed bananas, and then adjust accordingly the next time.

⟲ SWAP Prune puree *for* butter

Puree ½ cup of pitted prunes with ¼ cup of water in a blender or processor until smooth. The dark color and strong flavor of this fat substitute make it best suited for chocolate-based or heavily spiced baked goods, such as cookies, muffins, and quick breads. To replace 1 stick (½ cup) of butter, use ⅓ cup of prune puree.

⟲ SWAP Stevia *for* sugar

Stevia, a zero-calorie sweetener, is up to 300 times sweeter than sugar. I usually use only a few drops of liquid stevia in place of sugar in smoothies. If you overdo it, the taste becomes bitter, so start with a little and taste as you go.

⟲ SWAP Dates *for* sugar

Although dates are high in natural sugar, they're considered a low-glycemic-index food, meaning they won't spike your blood sugar. Medjool dates are my favorite because they're moist. Look for dates that are plump and free of crystallized sugar on the skins. To cook with them, soak them in hot water, and then remove the pits. Puree to use in smoothies, muffins, quick breads, pie fillings, or salad dressings.

⟲ SWAP Fat-free frozen yogurt *for* ice cream

When I want to enjoy a dessert à la mode or whip up a low-fat milk shake, I always opt for fat-free frozen yogurt. Look for brands that have live active cultures for an extra health boost (these beneficial bacteria have been shown to improve digestive health).

EVERYDAY SUPERFOODS

A superfood is one that's loaded with nutrition and significantly helps boost your health in some way. Although these foods offer big benefits, they don't cost big bucks. Plus, they're easy to find—many of these health-promoting picks are available at your local grocery store or farmers market—and incorporate into your diet. Here is a list of some of my favorite superfoods and information on how they keep you healthy from my friend, nutritionist Heather K. Jones; keep a lookout throughout the journal for superfood tips and recipes that use them:

----

❶ Blueberries

They may be small, but blueberries are nutritional powerhouses, packed with compounds that can help protect your heart, brain, eyes, and more. Blueberries contain polyphenols, which have antioxidant and anti-inflammatory properties that can ward off diseases like diabetes, cancer, and heart disease.

❷ Kiwifruit

One fuzzy fruit will nearly cover your daily vitamin C needs, is a great source of potassium, and is loaded with other good-for-you nutrients including folate, magnesium and the phytochemical lutein, which helps protect your eyes. One study even found that the compounds in kiwifruit may help improve sleep.

❸ Oranges

This citrus fruit offers 3 grams of filling fiber, nearly all the vitamin C you need in a day, some vitamin A, and folate. In a study from researchers in the United Kingdom, women who ate the most citrus fruits, which are rich in the antioxidant flavanones, had a lower risk for stroke than women who consumed the least.

❹ Mushrooms

Loaded with fiber, selenium, B vitamins, and potassium, mushrooms have been shown to help protect against cancer. They can also be a good source of vitamin D, which promotes bone health and may play a role in the prevention of a variety of diseases, including heart disease. And with so many varieties to choose from—

portobello, shiitake, morel, or white button, to name just a few—you're sure to find one that works in your favorite dishes.

❺ Cherries
Sure, cherries help make a mean pie, but they're so much more than simply pie filler. The little red orbs contain melatonin, the hormone that helps with sleep and may protect against some diseases. And their antioxidant and anti-inflammatory powers, courtesy of the fruits' anthocyanins, rival some of our best medicines—one study suggests cherries relieve pain better than aspirin.

❻ Sweet potatoes
One sweet potato contains nearly 4 grams of fiber and covers your daily vitamin A requirements. It also chips in some vitamin C, potassium, iron, and magnesium. The orange spud is a super source of beta-carotene, an antioxidant that may reduce the risk for cancer. Another benefit of beta-carotene: It can protect your skin from aging and damage and give you a healthy glow.

❼ Eggs
Eggs have gotten a bad rep over the years, but both egg whites and yolks contain healthful nutrients. The whites are a source of lean protein—there are 0 grams of saturated fat per a 3-ounce serving. And the yolks are a rich source of the antioxidants lutein and zeaxanthin, both of which help protect the eyes. Although the yolks are high in dietary cholesterol, one study found that people who ate one egg a day for five weeks had higher antioxidant levels without seeing any increases in cholesterol.

❽ Walnuts
On those days when you feel like a nut, it may be worth it to go for walnuts. In a study from the University of Pennsylvania, researchers found that walnuts had more (and higher quality) antioxidants than other nuts. Walnuts also contain the plant source of omega-3 fats called alpha-Linolenic acids (ALAs), which can help protect your heart, brain, and more.

❾ Broccoli
A member of the cruciferous family like its cauliflower cousin, broccoli is a good source of fiber, calcium, folate, and vitamins A, C, and K. It's also packed with potent disease-fighting antioxidants, such as

sulforaphane, kaempferol, quercetin, lutein, and zeaxanthin. Studies show that people who eat more broccoli have a lower risk for cancer.

⑩ Salmon

Need a reason to go fish? Here are some benefits to reeling in salmon: The fish is a source of lean protein and contains omega-3 fats, which prevent plaque formation in the arteries, reduce blood pressure, and decrease levels of triglycerides, a harmful fat found in the blood. For these reasons, the American Heart Association and other health groups recommend eating salmon and other fatty fish at least twice per week.

⑪ Yogurt

Yogurt can be a great source of protein, which is more satiating than fat and carbs. It's also loaded with calcium—an 8-ounce container covers nearly half of your daily needs for the bone-building mineral—and other vitamins and minerals. Some yogurt varieties earn extra points because they contain live active cultures of good bacteria, which have been shown to boost gut health. Be sure to steer clear of sweetened or flavored yogurts, which are more like desserts.

⑫ Kale

A good general nutrition guideline to keep in mind when produce shopping: The darker the color, the more antioxidants the fruit or vegetable usually contains. Perhaps that's why kale is so loaded with good-for-you compounds—including the phytochemicals lutein, zeaxanthin, beta-carotene, quercetin, and kaempferol—which have been shown to protect against cancer and other diseases. The dark leafy green also delivers a dose of vitamins A, C, and K, calcium and magnesium.

⑬ Apples

Apples have been shown to help reduce the risk for heart disease, cancer, asthma, and Alzheimer's. They may also help improve cognitive function, diabetes, weight control, and gut health. This may be because apples are rich in polyphenols, powerful antioxidants, and fiber, and also chip in some vitamin C and potassium. Enjoy them as a healthy snack, bake them into delicious desserts, have them as a savory side dish, or add them to your salad for a crunchy topping. How about them apples!

⓮ Flaxseeds

Flaxseeds are rich in fiber, ALAs (the plant form of omega-3 fatty acids), and lignans (plant compounds that act as antioxidants and phytoestrogens—a weaker form of the hormone estrogen—in the body). Research suggests that flaxseeds may help lower levels of A1C, a measure of blood sugar over three months, in people with diabetes. It may also reduce cholesterol in people with high cholesterol and help improve kidney function in people with lupus. In addition, flaxseeds seem to have some potential to fight prostate cancer.

⓯ Dark chocolate

Talk about sweet news—dark chocolate has been shown to protect the heart by lowering blood pressure, improving blood flow, and making platelets less sticky. Dark chocolate is made from cocoa, which contains flavonols, the same beneficial compounds found in grapes and wine. (Research suggests that dark chocolate has more antioxidants than milk or white chocolate.) Worried about your waistline? One study indicates that frequent chocolate eaters had a lower body mass index (a ratio of height to weight) than those who didn't enjoy chocolate regularly.

⓰ Green tea

It's tea time! Green tea is rich in antioxidants that may reduce your risk for diabetes, heart disease, and other conditions. One study found that those who drank six or more cups of green tea per day were 33 percent less likely to develop type 2 diabetes compared with those who drank less than one cup per day. Other research shows that people who drank green tea regularly for 10 years had less body fat and a smaller waist circumference than those who didn't. You can opt for regular green tea leaves or bags, or try the powdered form, called Matcha, to brew your own cup.

⓱ Garlic

This odorous vegetable may help with a number of conditions: Studies suggest that garlic may help reduce blood pressure by up to 8 percent in people with high blood pressure. It may also help keep arteries healthy and protect against a variety of cancers, including those of the colon, stomach, and rectum. The chemical that gives garlic its smell—allicin—also seems to be responsible for many of these health benefits.

18 Olive oil

Not all fats are created equal—there are good fats and then there are bad fats. Olive oil, without question, is a good fat. The oil, which is high in monounsaturated fat, the type that's heart-healthy, is a staple of the Mediterranean Diet, the eating style that is credited for the good health and longevity of the people living in that area. The benefits are numerous: Olive oil helps you feel full, protects against Alzheimer's, keeps your heart healthy, and boosts your brain power, to name just a few.

19 Avocados

Whether they're eaten plain, subbed for spreads like mayonnaise, mashed into guacamole, or used in a savory recipe, avocados are one of nature's finest—and most misunderstood—fruits. Historically slammed for their fat content, avocados are now lauded for their *beneficial* monounsaturated fats and omega-3s, which contribute to healthy cholesterol levels, prevent heart disease, and help us absorb the fat-soluble vitamins in the foods we pair with them. When selecting a ripe avocado, look for fruits that are firm and heavy and yield to gentle pressure without denting.

20 Tomatoes

No matter how you say it, tomatoes are nutrition superstars, thanks to their high content of lycopene. This antioxidant has been shown to help protect against a variety of cancers, osteoporosis, heart disease, and more. And unlike other compounds, lycopene is more easily absorbed by the body when it's cooked, so tomato products like sauce may offer even more antioxidants than raw tomatoes.

Food and Exercise Tracker

Track and plan your meals and exercise goals for the week.

Weekly Meal Planner

Weekly Goals _____

_____

_____

_____

_____

MON

TUE

WED

THU

FRI

SAT

SUN

Calories/Points Tracker

DAILY GOAL

MON	FOODS	CALORIES/POINTS	FOODS	CALORIES/POINTS
	B_____ ____		D_____ ____	
	_____ ____		_____ ____	
	_____ ____		_____ ____	
	_____ ____		_____ ____	
	_____ ____		_____ ____	
	_____ ____			
	L_____ ____		S_____ ____	
	_____ ____		_____ ____	
	_____ ____		_____ ____	
	_____ ____		_____ ____	
	_____ ____		_____ ____	
	_____ ____		TOTAL CALORIES/POINTS ____	

TUE	FOODS	CALORIES/POINTS	FOODS	CALORIES/POINTS
	B_____ ____		D_____ ____	
	_____ ____		_____ ____	
	_____ ____		_____ ____	
	_____ ____		_____ ____	
	_____ ____		_____ ____	
	_____ ____			
	L_____ ____		S_____ ____	
	_____ ____		_____ ____	
	_____ ____		_____ ____	
	_____ ____		_____ ____	
	_____ ____		_____ ____	
	_____ ____		TOTAL CALORIES/POINTS ____	

WED

FOODS	CALORIES/POINTS
B_____	___
_____	___
_____	___
_____	___
_____	___
_____	___
L_____	___
_____	___
_____	___
_____	___
_____	___
_____	___

FOODS	CALORIES/POINTS
D_____	___
_____	___
_____	___
_____	___
_____	___
_____	___
S_____	___
_____	___
_____	___
_____	___
TOTAL CALORIES/POINTS ___	

THU

FOODS	CALORIES/POINTS
B_____	___
_____	___
_____	___
_____	___
_____	___
_____	___
L_____	___
_____	___
_____	___
_____	___
_____	___
_____	___

FOODS	CALORIES/POINTS
D_____	___
_____	___
_____	___
_____	___
_____	___
_____	___
S_____	___
_____	___
_____	___
_____	___
TOTAL CALORIES/POINTS ___	

Calories/Points Tracker

DAILY GOAL _____

FRI

FOODS	CALORIES/POINTS	FOODS	CALORIES/POINTS
B_____	_____	D_____	_____
_____	_____	_____	_____
_____	_____	_____	_____
_____	_____	_____	_____
_____	_____	_____	_____
_____	_____	_____	_____
L_____	_____	S_____	_____
_____	_____	_____	_____
_____	_____	_____	_____
_____	_____	_____	_____
_____	_____	TOTAL CALORIES/POINTS	_____

SAT

FOODS	CALORIES/POINTS	FOODS	CALORIES/POINTS
B_____	_____	D_____	_____
_____	_____	_____	_____
_____	_____	_____	_____
_____	_____	_____	_____
_____	_____	_____	_____
_____	_____	_____	_____
L_____	_____	S_____	_____
_____	_____	_____	_____
_____	_____	_____	_____
_____	_____	_____	_____
_____	_____	TOTAL CALORIES/POINTS	_____

SUN

FOODS	CALORIES/ POINTS	FOODS	CALORIES/ POINTS
B_____	____	D_____	____
_____	____	_____	____
_____	____	_____	____
_____	____	_____	____
_____	____	_____	____
_____	____	_____	____
L_____	____	S_____	____
_____	____	_____	____
_____	____	_____	____
_____	____	_____	____
_____	____	TOTAL CALORIES/POINTS ____	
_____	____		

— Exercise Tracker —

ACTIVITY	DISTANCE/ DURATION/INTENSITY	CALORIES BURNED
_____	_____	_____
_____	_____	_____
_____	_____	_____
_____	_____	_____
_____	_____	_____
_____	_____	_____
_____	_____	_____
_____	_____	_____

Weekly Meal Planner

Weekly Goals _____

_____

_____

_____

_____

MON

TUE

WED

DATE ___/___/___ TO ___/___/___

THU

FRI

SAT

SUN

Calories/Points Tracker

DAILY GOAL

MON

FOODS	CALORIES/POINTS
B_____	_____
_____	_____
_____	_____
_____	_____
_____	_____
_____	_____
L_____	_____
_____	_____
_____	_____
_____	_____
_____	_____
_____	_____

FOODS	CALORIES/POINTS
D_____	_____
_____	_____
_____	_____
_____	_____
_____	_____
_____	_____
S_____	_____
_____	_____
_____	_____
_____	_____
TOTAL CALORIES/POINTS	_____

TUE

FOODS	CALORIES/POINTS
B_____	_____
_____	_____
_____	_____
_____	_____
_____	_____
_____	_____
L_____	_____
_____	_____
_____	_____
_____	_____
_____	_____
_____	_____

FOODS	CALORIES/POINTS
D_____	_____
_____	_____
_____	_____
_____	_____
_____	_____
_____	_____
S_____	_____
_____	_____
_____	_____
_____	_____
TOTAL CALORIES/POINTS	_____

DATE ___ / ___ / ___ TO ___ / ___ / ___

WED

FOODS	CALORIES/ POINTS	FOODS	CALORIES/ POINTS
B _____	_____	D _____	_____
_____	_____	_____	_____
_____	_____	_____	_____
_____	_____	_____	_____
_____	_____	_____	_____
_____	_____	_____	_____
L _____	_____	S _____	_____
_____	_____	_____	_____
_____	_____	_____	_____
_____	_____	_____	_____
_____	_____		
_____	_____	TOTAL CALORIES/POINTS _____

THU

FOODS	CALORIES/ POINTS	FOODS	CALORIES/ POINTS
B _____	_____	D _____	_____
_____	_____	_____	_____
_____	_____	_____	_____
_____	_____	_____	_____
_____	_____	_____	_____
_____	_____	_____	_____
L _____	_____	S _____	_____
_____	_____	_____	_____
_____	_____	_____	_____
_____	_____	_____	_____
_____	_____		
_____	_____	TOTAL CALORIES/POINTS _____

Calories/Points Tracker

FRI

FOODS   CALORIES/POINTS

B _____ _____
_____ _____
_____ _____
_____ _____
_____ _____
_____ _____

L _____ _____
_____ _____
_____ _____
_____ _____
_____ _____
_____ _____

FOODS   CALORIES/POINTS

D _____ _____
_____ _____
_____ _____
_____ _____
_____ _____
_____ _____

S _____ _____
_____ _____
_____ _____
_____ _____

TOTAL CALORIES/POINTS _____

SAT

FOODS   CALORIES/POINTS

B _____ _____
_____ _____
_____ _____
_____ _____
_____ _____
_____ _____

L _____ _____
_____ _____
_____ _____
_____ _____
_____ _____
_____ _____

FOODS   CALORIES/POINTS

D _____ _____
_____ _____
_____ _____
_____ _____
_____ _____
_____ _____

S _____ _____
_____ _____
_____ _____
_____ _____

TOTAL CALORIES/POINTS _____

SUN

FOODS	CALORIES/ POINTS	FOODS	CALORIES/ POINTS
B_____ _____		D_____ _____	
_____ _____		_____ _____	
_____ _____		_____ _____	
_____ _____		_____ _____	
_____ _____		_____ _____	
_____ _____		_____ _____	
L_____ _____		S_____ _____	
_____ _____		_____ _____	
_____ _____		_____ _____	
_____ _____		_____ _____	
_____ _____			
_____ _____		TOTAL CALORIES/POINTS _____	

—————————————— Exercise Tracker ——————————————

ACTIVITY	DISTANCE/ DURATION/INTENSITY	CALORIES BURNED
_____	_____	_____
_____	_____	_____
_____	_____	_____
_____	_____	_____
_____	_____	_____
_____	_____	_____
_____	_____	_____
_____	_____	_____

Weekly Meal Planner

Weekly Goals _____

_____

_____

_____

_____

MON

_____

_____

_____

_____

_____

TUE

_____

_____

_____

_____

_____

WED

_____

_____

_____

_____

_____

DATE ___/___/___ TO ___/___/___

THU

FRI

SAT

SUN

Calories/Points Tracker

MON

FOODS	CALORIES/ POINTS
B	
L	

FOODS	CALORIES/ POINTS
D	
S	

TOTAL CALORIES/POINTS _____

TUE

FOODS	CALORIES/ POINTS
B	
L	

FOODS	CALORIES/ POINTS
D	
S	

TOTAL CALORIES/POINTS _____

WED

FOODS	CALORIES/POINTS	FOODS	CALORIES/POINTS
B_____	_____	D_____	_____
_____	_____	_____	_____
_____	_____	_____	_____
_____	_____	_____	_____
_____	_____	_____	_____
_____	_____	_____	_____
L_____	_____	S_____	_____
_____	_____	_____	_____
_____	_____	_____	_____
_____	_____	_____	_____
_____	_____		
_____	_____	TOTAL CALORIES/POINTS _____	

THU

FOODS	CALORIES/POINTS	FOODS	CALORIES/POINTS
B_____	_____	D_____	_____
_____	_____	_____	_____
_____	_____	_____	_____
_____	_____	_____	_____
_____	_____	_____	_____
_____	_____	_____	_____
L_____	_____	S_____	_____
_____	_____	_____	_____
_____	_____	_____	_____
_____	_____	_____	_____
_____	_____		
_____	_____	TOTAL CALORIES/POINTS _____	

Calories/Points Tracker

FRI

FOODS	CALORIES/POINTS	FOODS	CALORIES/POINTS
B_____	_____	D_____	_____
_____	_____	_____	_____
_____	_____	_____	_____
_____	_____	_____	_____
_____	_____	_____	_____
_____	_____	_____	_____
L_____	_____	S_____	_____
_____	_____	_____	_____
_____	_____	_____	_____
_____	_____	_____	_____
_____	_____	_____	_____
_____	_____	TOTAL CALORIES/POINTS	_____

SAT

FOODS	CALORIES/POINTS	FOODS	CALORIES/POINTS
B_____	_____	D_____	_____
_____	_____	_____	_____
_____	_____	_____	_____
_____	_____	_____	_____
_____	_____	_____	_____
_____	_____	_____	_____
L_____	_____	S_____	_____
_____	_____	_____	_____
_____	_____	_____	_____
_____	_____	_____	_____
_____	_____	_____	_____
_____	_____	TOTAL CALORIES/POINTS	_____

SUN

DATE ___ / ___ / ___ TO ___ / ___ / ___

FOODS	CALORIES/POINTS	FOODS	CALORIES/POINTS
B_____	_____	D_____	_____
_____	_____	_____	_____
_____	_____	_____	_____
_____	_____	_____	_____
_____	_____	_____	_____
_____	_____	_____	_____
L_____	_____	S_____	_____
_____	_____	_____	_____
_____	_____	_____	_____
_____	_____	_____	_____
_____	_____		
_____	_____	TOTAL CALORIES/POINTS _____	

―――――――― Exercise Tracker ――――――――

ACTIVITY	DISTANCE/DURATION/INTENSITY	CALORIES BURNED
_____	_____	_____
_____	_____	_____
_____	_____	_____
_____	_____	_____
_____	_____	_____
_____	_____	_____
_____	_____	_____
_____	_____	_____

Blueberry-Banana-Oatmeal Smoothie

MAKES 3½ CUPS; SERVES 2

2 cups water

½ cup raw quick oats*

½ cup unsweetened vanilla almond milk (I like Almond Breeze)

½ cup blueberries, fresh or frozen

½ ripe medium banana

½ teaspoon vanilla extract

2 tablespoons raw sugar

½ cup ice

In a small saucepan set over medium heat, bring the water to a boil. Add the oats and cook, stirring often, until thick and bubbly, 1 to 2 minutes. Let cool for a few minutes.

In a blender, combine the cooled oats, almond milk, blueberries, banana, vanilla extract, sugar, and ice. Blend on high until very smooth. Pour in a glass filled with ice and serve.

*Use gluten-free oats to make this gluten-free.

SERVING SIZE	1¾ cup
CALORIES	179
FAT	2 g
CHOLESTEROL	0 mg
CARBOHYDRATE	38 g
FIBER	4 g
PROTEIN	3 g
SUGAR	8 g
SODIUM	52.5 mg

Frozen Mango-Kiwifruit-Raspberry Pops

MAKES 4 POPS

9 tablespoons water

2 tablespoons sugar

5 ounces peeled kiwifruit

6 ounces peeled mango

6 ounces fresh raspberries

SERVING SIZE	1 pop
CALORIES	91.5
FAT	0.5 g
CHOLESTEROL	0 mg
CARBOHYDRATE	22 g
FIBER	4 g
PROTEIN	1 g
SUGAR	12 g
SODIUM	1.8 mg

Make a simple syrup by bringing the water and sugar to a boil in a small pot set over medium heat. Cook until syrupy, 4 to 5 minutes. Set aside.

Puree the fruit separately in a blender. Transfer to three small bowls. Divide the simple syrup among the fruit purees and stir well.

Divide the kiwifruit puree among four small (5-ounce) cups and freeze for 1 hour.

Remove from the freezer and divide the mango puree over the kiwifruit puree. Freeze for 20 minutes. Remove from the freezer, insert sticks, and freeze at least 2 hours.

Remove from the freezer, divide the raspberry puree over the mango puree, and freeze overnight.

Weekly Meal Planner

Weekly Goals _____

_____

_____

_____

_____

_____

> "Do one thing
> every day that
> scares you."
>
> MARY SCHMICH

MON

TUE

WED

THU

FRI

SAT

SUN

Calories/Points Tracker

MON

FOODS	CALORIES/ POINTS
B _____	_____
_____	_____
_____	_____
_____	_____
_____	_____
L _____	_____
_____	_____
_____	_____
_____	_____
_____	_____

FOODS	CALORIES/ POINTS
D _____	_____
_____	_____
_____	_____
_____	_____
_____	_____
S _____	_____
_____	_____
_____	_____
_____	_____
TOTAL CALORIES/POINTS	_____

TUE

FOODS	CALORIES/ POINTS
B _____	_____
_____	_____
_____	_____
_____	_____
_____	_____
L _____	_____
_____	_____
_____	_____
_____	_____
_____	_____

FOODS	CALORIES/ POINTS
D _____	_____
_____	_____
_____	_____
_____	_____
_____	_____
S _____	_____
_____	_____
_____	_____
_____	_____
TOTAL CALORIES/POINTS	_____

DATE ___/___/___ TO ___/___/___

FOODS	CALORIES/POINTS	FOODS	CALORIES/POINTS
B_____	_____	D_____	_____
_____	_____	_____	_____
_____	_____	_____	_____
_____	_____	_____	_____
_____	_____	_____	_____
_____	_____	_____	_____
L_____	_____	S_____	_____
_____	_____	_____	_____
_____	_____	_____	_____
_____	_____	_____	_____
_____	_____		
_____	_____	TOTAL CALORIES/POINTS _____	

FOODS	CALORIES/POINTS	FOODS	CALORIES/POINTS
B_____	_____	D_____	_____
_____	_____	_____	_____
_____	_____	_____	_____
_____	_____	_____	_____
_____	_____	_____	_____
_____	_____	_____	_____
L_____	_____	S_____	_____
_____	_____	_____	_____
_____	_____	_____	_____
_____	_____	_____	_____
_____	_____		
_____	_____	TOTAL CALORIES/POINTS _____	

Calories/Points Tracker

DAILY GOAL

FOODS	CALORIES/ POINTS	FOODS	CALORIES/ POINTS
B _____	_____	D _____	_____
_____	_____	_____	_____
_____	_____	_____	_____
_____	_____	_____	_____
_____	_____	_____	_____
_____	_____	_____	_____
L _____	_____	S _____	_____
_____	_____	_____	_____
_____	_____	_____	_____
_____	_____	_____	_____
_____	_____	TOTAL CALORIES/POINTS	_____

FRI

FOODS	CALORIES/ POINTS	FOODS	CALORIES/ POINTS
B _____	_____	D _____	_____
_____	_____	_____	_____
_____	_____	_____	_____
_____	_____	_____	_____
_____	_____	_____	_____
_____	_____	_____	_____
L _____	_____	S _____	_____
_____	_____	_____	_____
_____	_____	_____	_____
_____	_____	_____	_____
_____	_____	TOTAL CALORIES/POINTS	_____

SAT

DATE ___ / ___ / ___ TO ___ / ___ / ___

FOODS	CALORIES/POINTS	FOODS	CALORIES/POINTS
B_____	___	D_____	___
_____	___	_____	___
_____	___	_____	___
_____	___	_____	___
_____	___	_____	___
_____	___	_____	___
L_____	___	S_____	___
_____	___	_____	___
_____	___	_____	___
_____	___	_____	___
_____	___	TOTAL CALORIES/POINTS	___

— Exercise Tracker —

ACTIVITY	DISTANCE/DURATION/INTENSITY	CALORIES BURNED
_____	_____	_____
_____	_____	_____
_____	_____	_____
_____	_____	_____
_____	_____	_____
_____	_____	_____
_____	_____	_____

Weekly Meal Planner

Weekly Goals _____

_____

_____

_____

_____

superfood

KIWIFRUIT

This small fuzzy fruit is pleasingly tart and has little seeds inside that are fun to crunch. Slice one into a fruit salad, or even scoop the flesh from the skin with a spoon for a snack!

MON

TUE

WED

THU

FRI

SAT

SUN

Calories/Points Tracker

DAILY GOAL

MON

FOODS	CALORIES/POINTS	FOODS	CALORIES/POINTS
B _____	_____	D _____	_____
_____	_____	_____	_____
_____	_____	_____	_____
_____	_____	_____	_____
_____	_____	_____	_____
_____	_____	_____	_____
L _____	_____	S _____	_____
_____	_____	_____	_____
_____	_____	_____	_____
_____	_____	_____	_____
_____	_____	TOTAL CALORIES/POINTS _____	

TUE

FOODS	CALORIES/POINTS	FOODS	CALORIES/POINTS
B _____	_____	D _____	_____
_____	_____	_____	_____
_____	_____	_____	_____
_____	_____	_____	_____
_____	_____	_____	_____
_____	_____	_____	_____
L _____	_____	S _____	_____
_____	_____	_____	_____
_____	_____	_____	_____
_____	_____	_____	_____
_____	_____	TOTAL CALORIES/POINTS _____	

WED

FOODS	CALORIES/POINTS	FOODS	CALORIES/POINTS
B_____	_____	D_____	_____
_____	_____	_____	_____
_____	_____	_____	_____
_____	_____	_____	_____
_____	_____	_____	_____
_____	_____	_____	_____
L_____	_____	S_____	_____
_____	_____	_____	_____
_____	_____	_____	_____
_____	_____	_____	_____
_____	_____	TOTAL CALORIES/POINTS _____

THU

FOODS	CALORIES/POINTS	FOODS	CALORIES/POINTS
B_____	_____	D_____	_____
_____	_____	_____	_____
_____	_____	_____	_____
_____	_____	_____	_____
_____	_____	_____	_____
_____	_____	_____	_____
L_____	_____	S_____	_____
_____	_____	_____	_____
_____	_____	_____	_____
_____	_____	_____	_____
_____	_____	TOTAL CALORIES/POINTS _____

Calories/Points Tracker

DAILY GOAL

FRI

FOODS	CALORIES/POINTS
B_____	_____
_____	_____
_____	_____
_____	_____
_____	_____
_____	_____
L_____	_____
_____	_____
_____	_____
_____	_____
_____	_____
_____	_____

FOODS	CALORIES/POINTS
D_____	_____
_____	_____
_____	_____
_____	_____
_____	_____
S_____	_____
_____	_____
_____	_____
_____	_____
TOTAL CALORIES/POINTS	_____

SAT

FOODS	CALORIES/POINTS
B_____	_____
_____	_____
_____	_____
_____	_____
_____	_____
_____	_____
L_____	_____
_____	_____
_____	_____
_____	_____
_____	_____
_____	_____

FOODS	CALORIES/POINTS
D_____	_____
_____	_____
_____	_____
_____	_____
_____	_____
S_____	_____
_____	_____
_____	_____
_____	_____
TOTAL CALORIES/POINTS	_____

DATE ___/___/___ TO ___/___/___

SUN

FOODS	CALORIES/POINTS	FOODS	CALORIES/POINTS
B_____	_____	D_____	_____
_____	_____	_____	_____
_____	_____	_____	_____
_____	_____	_____	_____
_____	_____	_____	_____
_____	_____	_____	_____
L_____	_____	S_____	_____
_____	_____	_____	_____
_____	_____	_____	_____
_____	_____	_____	_____
_____	_____		
_____	_____	TOTAL CALORIES/POINTS _____	

—————————————— Exercise Tracker ——————————————

ACTIVITY	DISTANCE/DURATION/INTENSITY	CALORIES BURNED
_____	_____	_____
_____	_____	_____
_____	_____	_____
_____	_____	_____
_____	_____	_____
_____	_____	_____
_____	_____	_____

Weekly Meal Planner

Weekly Goals _____

_____

_____

_____

_____

> "It does not matter
> how slowly you
> go as long as you
> do not stop."
>
> ——————
> **CONFUCIUS**

MON

_____

_____

_____

_____

TUE

_____

_____

_____

_____

WED

_____

_____

_____

_____

THU

FRI

SAT

SUN

Calories/Points Tracker

DAILY GOAL _____

MON

FOODS	CALORIES/POINTS
B_____	____
_____	____
_____	____
_____	____
_____	____
_____	____
L_____	____
_____	____
_____	____
_____	____
_____	____
_____	____

FOODS	CALORIES/POINTS
D_____	____
_____	____
_____	____
_____	____
_____	____
S_____	____
_____	____
_____	____
_____	____
TOTAL CALORIES/POINTS	____

TUE

FOODS	CALORIES/POINTS
B_____	____
_____	____
_____	____
_____	____
_____	____
_____	____
L_____	____
_____	____
_____	____
_____	____
_____	____
_____	____

FOODS	CALORIES/POINTS
D_____	____
_____	____
_____	____
_____	____
_____	____
S_____	____
_____	____
_____	____
_____	____
TOTAL CALORIES/POINTS	____

DATE ___/___/___ TO ___/___/___

FOODS	CALORIES/POINTS	FOODS	CALORIES/POINTS
B _____	_____	D _____	_____
_____	_____	_____	_____
_____	_____	_____	_____
_____	_____	_____	_____
_____	_____	_____	_____
_____	_____	_____	_____
L _____	_____	S _____	_____
_____	_____	_____	_____
_____	_____	_____	_____
_____	_____	_____	_____
_____	_____	TOTAL CALORIES/POINTS _____
_____	_____		

FOODS	CALORIES/POINTS	FOODS	CALORIES/POINTS
B _____	_____	D _____	_____
_____	_____	_____	_____
_____	_____	_____	_____
_____	_____	_____	_____
_____	_____	_____	_____
_____	_____	_____	_____
L _____	_____	S _____	_____
_____	_____	_____	_____
_____	_____	_____	_____
_____	_____	_____	_____
_____	_____	TOTAL CALORIES/POINTS _____

Calories/Points Tracker

DAILY GOAL _____

FRI

FOODS	CALORIES/POINTS	FOODS	CALORIES/POINTS
B _____	____	D _____	____
_____	____	_____	____
_____	____	_____	____
_____	____	_____	____
_____	____	_____	____
L _____	____	S _____	____
_____	____	_____	____
_____	____	_____	____
_____	____	_____	____
_____	____	TOTAL CALORIES/POINTS ____	

SAT

FOODS	CALORIES/POINTS	FOODS	CALORIES/POINTS
B _____	____	D _____	____
_____	____	_____	____
_____	____	_____	____
_____	____	_____	____
_____	____	_____	____
L _____	____	S _____	____
_____	____	_____	____
_____	____	_____	____
_____	____	_____	____
_____	____	TOTAL CALORIES/POINTS ____	

DATE ___ / ___ / ___ TO ___ / ___ / ___

FOODS	CALORIES/POINTS	FOODS	CALORIES/POINTS
B_____	_____	D_____	_____
_____	_____	_____	_____
_____	_____	_____	_____
_____	_____	_____	_____
_____	_____	_____	_____
_____	_____	_____	_____
L_____	_____	S_____	_____
_____	_____	_____	_____
_____	_____	_____	_____
_____	_____	_____	_____
_____	_____	TOTAL CALORIES/POINTS _____	

—————— Exercise Tracker ——————

ACTIVITY	DISTANCE/DURATION/INTENSITY	CALORIES BURNED
_____	_____	_____
_____	_____	_____
_____	_____	_____
_____	_____	_____
_____	_____	_____
_____	_____	_____
_____	_____	_____
_____	_____	_____

Orange, Red Onion, Gorgonzola, and Arugula Salad

MAKES 1 SALAD; SERVES 1

- 1 small orange, peeled and sectioned
- 1 teaspoon balsamic vinegar
- 1 teaspoon extra-virgin olive oil
- ½ teaspoon honey
- ⅛ teaspoon kosher salt
- Freshly ground black pepper

- 2 cups baby greens, such as arugula and spinach
- 3 tablespoons crumbled gorgonzola cheese, or other blue cheese
- 3 thin slices red onion

Take 2 sections of the orange and squeeze the juice into a small bowl. Whisk in the vinegar, oil, honey, and salt, and season with pepper.

Arrange the baby greens on a plate. Cut the remaining orange sections into bite-size pieces and scatter them over the greens. Scatter the cheese and red onion over the salad. Drizzle the vinaigrette over the top and serve.

SERVING SIZE	1 salad
CALORIES	246
FAT	13.5 g
CHOLESTEROL	30 mg
CARBOHYDRATE	22 g
FIBER	4 g
PROTEIN	10 g
SUGAR	14 g
SODIUM	567 mg

Easy Garden Tomato Sauce

MAKES 2½ CUPS; SERVES 5

1 tablespoon olive oil

6 garlic cloves, chopped

1½ pounds grape tomatoes, cut in half

⅛ teaspoon crushed red pepper flakes

¾ teaspoon kosher salt

Freshly ground black pepper

2 tablespoons chopped fresh oregano, or chopped fresh basil

In a large nonstick pan set over high heat, heat the oil. Add the garlic and cook until golden, 30 seconds. Add the tomatoes, crushed red pepper flakes, and salt, and season with pepper. Reduce the heat to low. Simmer, covered, until the tomatoes soften, 15 minutes. Stir in the oregano and cook 15 more minutes.

SERVING SIZE	½ cup
CALORIES	58
FAT	3 g
CHOLESTEROL	0 mg
CARBOHYDRATE	7.5 g
FIBER	1.6 g
PROTEIN	1.5 g
SUGAR	0 g
SODIUM	181 mg

Weekly Meal Planner

Weekly Goals _____

_____

_____

_____

_____

superfood

ORANGES

Widely available, this citrus is a great addition to a salad, and it's sweet enough to stand in for dessert.

MON

_____

_____

_____

_____

TUE

_____

_____

_____

_____

WED

_____

_____

_____

_____

DATE ___/___/___ TO ___/___/___

THU

FRI

SAT

SUN

Calories/Points Tracker

DAILY GOAL _____

MON

FOODS	CALORIES/POINTS	FOODS	CALORIES/POINTS
B_____	_____	D_____	_____
_____	_____	_____	_____
_____	_____	_____	_____
_____	_____	_____	_____
_____	_____	_____	_____
_____	_____	_____	_____
L_____	_____	S_____	_____
_____	_____	_____	_____
_____	_____	_____	_____
_____	_____	_____	_____
_____	_____		
_____	_____	TOTAL CALORIES/POINTS _____	

TUE

FOODS	CALORIES/POINTS	FOODS	CALORIES/POINTS
B_____	_____	D_____	_____
_____	_____	_____	_____
_____	_____	_____	_____
_____	_____	_____	_____
_____	_____	_____	_____
_____	_____	_____	_____
L_____	_____	S_____	_____
_____	_____	_____	_____
_____	_____	_____	_____
_____	_____	_____	_____
_____	_____		
_____	_____	TOTAL CALORIES/POINTS _____	

DATE _____ / _____ / _____ TO _____ / _____ / _____

FOODS	CALORIES/ POINTS	FOODS	CALORIES/ POINTS
B_____	____	D_____	____
_____	____	_____	____
_____	____	_____	____
_____	____	_____	____
_____	____	_____	____
_____	____	_____	____
L_____	____	S_____	____
_____	____	_____	____
_____	____	_____	____
_____	____	_____	____
_____	____	_____	____
_____	____	TOTAL CALORIES/POINTS ____	

FOODS	CALORIES/ POINTS	FOODS	CALORIES/ POINTS
B_____	____	D_____	____
_____	____	_____	____
_____	____	_____	____
_____	____	_____	____
_____	____	_____	____
_____	____	_____	____
L_____	____	S_____	____
_____	____	_____	____
_____	____	_____	____
_____	____	_____	____
_____	____	_____	____
_____	____	TOTAL CALORIES/POINTS ____	

Calories/Points Tracker

DAILY GOAL

FRI

FOODS	CALORIES/ POINTS	FOODS	CALORIES/ POINTS
B_____	_____	D_____	_____
_____	_____	_____	_____
_____	_____	_____	_____
_____	_____	_____	_____
_____	_____	_____	_____
_____	_____	S_____	_____
L_____	_____	_____	_____
_____	_____	_____	_____
_____	_____	_____	_____
_____	_____	_____	_____
_____	_____		
_____	_____	TOTAL CALORIES/POINTS _____	

SAT

FOODS	CALORIES/ POINTS	FOODS	CALORIES/ POINTS
B_____	_____	D_____	_____
_____	_____	_____	_____
_____	_____	_____	_____
_____	_____	_____	_____
_____	_____	_____	_____
L_____	_____	S_____	_____
_____	_____	_____	_____
_____	_____	_____	_____
_____	_____	_____	_____
_____	_____		
_____	_____	TOTAL CALORIES/POINTS _____	

DATE ___/___/___ TO ___/___/___

SUN

FOODS	CALORIES/ POINTS	FOODS	CALORIES/ POINTS
B_____	____	D_____	____
_____	____	_____	____
_____	____	_____	____
_____	____	_____	____
_____	____	_____	____
_____	____	_____	____
L_____	____	S_____	____
_____	____	_____	____
_____	____	_____	____
_____	____	_____	____
_____	____		
_____	____	TOTAL CALORIES/POINTS ____

———————————— Exercise Tracker ————————————

ACTIVITY	DISTANCE/ DURATION/INTENSITY	CALORIES BURNED
_____	_____	_____
_____	_____	_____
_____	_____	_____
_____	_____	_____
_____	_____	_____
_____	_____	_____
_____	_____	_____
_____	_____	_____

Weekly Meal Planner

Weekly Goals _____

_____

_____

_____

_____

> "Whether you
> believe you can
> do a thing or not,
> you are right."
>
> **HENRY FORD**

MON

_____

_____

_____

_____

TUE

_____

_____

_____

_____

WED

_____

_____

_____

_____

THU

FRI

SAT

SUN

Calories/Points Tracker

DAILY GOAL [ ]

MON

FOODS	CALORIES/POINTS	FOODS	CALORIES/POINTS
B_____	____	D_____	____
_____	____	_____	____
_____	____	_____	____
_____	____	_____	____
_____	____	_____	____
_____	____	_____	____
L_____	____	S_____	____
_____	____	_____	____
_____	____	_____	____
_____	____	_____	____
_____	____	_____	____
_____	____	TOTAL CALORIES/POINTS ____

TUE

FOODS	CALORIES/POINTS	FOODS	CALORIES/POINTS
B_____	____	D_____	____
_____	____	_____	____
_____	____	_____	____
_____	____	_____	____
_____	____	_____	____
_____	____	_____	____
L_____	____	S_____	____
_____	____	_____	____
_____	____	_____	____
_____	____	_____	____
_____	____	_____	____
_____	____	TOTAL CALORIES/POINTS ____

DATE ___ / ___ / ___ TO ___ / ___ / ___

FOODS	CALORIES/POINTS	FOODS	CALORIES/POINTS
B_____	_____	D_____	_____
_____	_____	_____	_____
_____	_____	_____	_____
_____	_____	_____	_____
_____	_____	_____	_____
_____	_____	_____	_____
L_____	_____	S_____	_____
_____	_____	_____	_____
_____	_____	_____	_____
_____	_____	_____	_____
_____	_____	TOTAL CALORIES/POINTS _____	

FOODS	CALORIES/POINTS	FOODS	CALORIES/POINTS
B_____	_____	D_____	_____
_____	_____	_____	_____
_____	_____	_____	_____
_____	_____	_____	_____
_____	_____	_____	_____
_____	_____	_____	_____
L_____	_____	S_____	_____
_____	_____	_____	_____
_____	_____	_____	_____
_____	_____	_____	_____
_____	_____	TOTAL CALORIES/POINTS _____	

Calories/Points Tracker

DAILY GOAL [   ]

FRI

FOODS	CALORIES/POINTS	FOODS	CALORIES/POINTS
B _____	_____	D _____	_____
_____	_____	_____	_____
_____	_____	_____	_____
_____	_____	_____	_____
_____	_____	_____	_____
_____	_____	_____	_____
L _____	_____	S _____	_____
_____	_____	_____	_____
_____	_____	_____	_____
_____	_____	_____	_____
_____	_____		
_____	_____	TOTAL CALORIES/POINTS	_____

SAT

FOODS	CALORIES/POINTS	FOODS	CALORIES/POINTS
B _____	_____	D _____	_____
_____	_____	_____	_____
_____	_____	_____	_____
_____	_____	_____	_____
_____	_____	_____	_____
_____	_____	_____	_____
L _____	_____	S _____	_____
_____	_____	_____	_____
_____	_____	_____	_____
_____	_____	_____	_____
_____	_____		
_____	_____	TOTAL CALORIES/POINTS	_____

DATE ___ / ___ / ___ TO ___ / ___ / ___

FOODS	CALORIES/ POINTS	FOODS	CALORIES/ POINTS
B_____	_____	D_____	_____
_____	_____	_____	_____
_____	_____	_____	_____
_____	_____	_____	_____
_____	_____	_____	_____
_____	_____	_____	_____
L_____	_____	S_____	_____
_____	_____	_____	_____
_____	_____	_____	_____
_____	_____	_____	_____
_____	_____		
_____	_____	TOTAL CALORIES/POINTS _____	

Exercise Tracker

ACTIVITY	DISTANCE/ DURATION/INTENSITY	CALORIES BURNED
_____	_____	_____
_____	_____	_____
_____	_____	_____
_____	_____	_____
_____	_____	_____
_____	_____	_____
_____	_____	_____
_____	_____	_____

Weekly Meal Planner

Weekly Goals _____

_____

_____

_____

_____

> "Success is not the key to happiness. Happiness is the key to success."
>
> **ALBERT SCHWEITZER**

MON

TUE

WED

THU

FRI

SAT

SUN

Calories/Points Tracker

DAILY GOAL

MON

FOODS	CALORIES/POINTS	FOODS	CALORIES/POINTS
B_____	_____	D_____	_____
_____	_____	_____	_____
_____	_____	_____	_____
_____	_____	_____	_____
_____	_____	_____	_____
_____	_____	_____	_____
L_____	_____	S_____	_____
_____	_____	_____	_____
_____	_____	_____	_____
_____	_____	_____	_____
_____	_____		
_____	_____	TOTAL CALORIES/POINTS _____	

TUE

FOODS	CALORIES/POINTS	FOODS	CALORIES/POINTS
B_____	_____	D_____	_____
_____	_____	_____	_____
_____	_____	_____	_____
_____	_____	_____	_____
_____	_____	_____	_____
_____	_____	_____	_____
L_____	_____	S_____	_____
_____	_____	_____	_____
_____	_____	_____	_____
_____	_____	_____	_____
_____	_____		
_____	_____	TOTAL CALORIES/POINTS _____	

DATE ____/____/____ TO ____/____/____

WED

FOODS	CALORIES/POINTS	FOODS	CALORIES/POINTS
B_____	_____	D_____	_____
_____	_____	_____	_____
_____	_____	_____	_____
_____	_____	_____	_____
_____	_____	_____	_____
_____	_____	_____	_____
L_____	_____	S_____	_____
_____	_____	_____	_____
_____	_____	_____	_____
_____	_____	_____	_____
_____	_____		
_____	_____	TOTAL CALORIES/POINTS _____	

THU

FOODS	CALORIES/POINTS	FOODS	CALORIES/POINTS
B_____	_____	D_____	_____
_____	_____	_____	_____
_____	_____	_____	_____
_____	_____	_____	_____
_____	_____	_____	_____
_____	_____	_____	_____
L_____	_____	S_____	_____
_____	_____	_____	_____
_____	_____	_____	_____
_____	_____	_____	_____
_____	_____		
_____	_____	TOTAL CALORIES/POINTS _____	

Calories/Points Tracker

DAILY GOAL _____

FRI

FOODS	CALORIES/POINTS	FOODS	CALORIES/POINTS
B _____	_____	D _____	_____
_____	_____	_____	_____
_____	_____	_____	_____
_____	_____	_____	_____
_____	_____	_____	_____
_____	_____	_____	_____
L _____	_____	S _____	_____
_____	_____	_____	_____
_____	_____	_____	_____
_____	_____	_____	_____
_____	_____	TOTAL CALORIES/POINTS	_____

SAT

FOODS	CALORIES/POINTS	FOODS	CALORIES/POINTS
B _____	_____	D _____	_____
_____	_____	_____	_____
_____	_____	_____	_____
_____	_____	_____	_____
_____	_____	_____	_____
_____	_____	_____	_____
L _____	_____	S _____	_____
_____	_____	_____	_____
_____	_____	_____	_____
_____	_____	_____	_____
_____	_____	TOTAL CALORIES/POINTS	_____

DATE ___ / ___ / ___ TO ___ / ___ / ___

SUN

FOODS	CALORIES/ POINTS	FOODS	CALORIES/ POINTS
B _____	_____	D _____	_____
_____	_____	_____	_____
_____	_____	_____	_____
_____	_____	_____	_____
_____	_____	_____	_____
_____	_____	_____	_____
L _____	_____	S _____	_____
_____	_____	_____	_____
_____	_____	_____	_____
_____	_____	_____	_____
_____	_____		
_____	_____	TOTAL CALORIES/POINTS _____	

—————— Exercise Tracker ——————

ACTIVITY	DISTANCE/ DURATION/INTENSITY	CALORIES BURNED
_____	_____	_____
_____	_____	_____
_____	_____	_____
_____	_____	_____
_____	_____	_____
_____	_____	_____
_____	_____	_____
_____	_____	_____

Cherry Custard

Nonstick cooking spray

¼ cup unbleached all-purpose flour, sifted, plus more for dusting

1⅓ cups pitted cherries, halved

¼ cup raw sugar

2 large eggs

Pinch of kosher salt

½ cup fat-free milk

1 teaspoon vanilla extract

Confectioners' sugar, for dusting (optional)

SERVING SIZE	1 custard
CALORIES	155
FAT	2.5 g
CHOLESTEROL	94 mg
CARBOHYDRATE	27.5 g
FIBER	1.3 g
PROTEIN	5.5 g
SUGAR	8 g
SODIUM	56.5 mg

Preheat the oven to 350°F. Lightly spray four 5-ounce ramekins with nonstick cooking spray and dust with a little flour. Divide the cherries among the ramekins.

In a medium bowl, whisk together the flour, sugar, eggs, and salt. Add the milk and vanilla extract, and whisk until smooth. Divide among the ramekins.

Bake until lightly browned and a toothpick inserted into the center comes out clean, 25 to 28 minutes. Transfer to a wire rack and let cool completely. (When you pull it out of the oven, it will wiggle and puff up, and then deflate while cooling.)

When cool, dust with confectioners' sugar, if using, and serve.

Weekly Meal Planner

Weekly Goals _____

_____

_____

_____

_____

superfood

MUSHROOMS

You will reap nutritional benefits from any type of mushroom. Sauté some until golden brown, and add to pastas, egg dishes, or serve as a side dish.

MON

TUE

WED

THU

FRI

SAT

SUN

Calories/Points Tracker

MON

FOODS CALORIES/POINTS

B _____ _____
_____ _____
_____ _____
_____ _____
_____ _____
_____ _____

L _____ _____
_____ _____
_____ _____
_____ _____
_____ _____

FOODS CALORIES/POINTS

D _____ _____
_____ _____
_____ _____
_____ _____
_____ _____

S _____ _____
_____ _____
_____ _____
_____ _____

TOTAL CALORIES/POINTS _____

TUE

FOODS CALORIES/POINTS

B _____ _____
_____ _____
_____ _____
_____ _____
_____ _____

L _____ _____
_____ _____
_____ _____
_____ _____
_____ _____

FOODS CALORIES/POINTS

D _____ _____
_____ _____
_____ _____
_____ _____
_____ _____

S _____ _____
_____ _____
_____ _____
_____ _____

TOTAL CALORIES/POINTS _____

WED

FOODS	CALORIES/POINTS	FOODS	CALORIES/POINTS
B_____ _____		D_____ _____	
_____ _____		_____ _____	
_____ _____		_____ _____	
_____ _____		_____ _____	
_____ _____		_____ _____	
_____ _____		_____ _____	
L_____ _____		S_____ _____	
_____ _____		_____ _____	
_____ _____		_____ _____	
_____ _____		_____ _____	
_____ _____			
_____ _____		TOTAL CALORIES/POINTS _____	

THU

FOODS	CALORIES/POINTS	FOODS	CALORIES/POINTS
B_____ _____		D_____ _____	
_____ _____		_____ _____	
_____ _____		_____ _____	
_____ _____		_____ _____	
_____ _____		_____ _____	
L_____ _____		_____ _____	
_____ _____		S_____ _____	
_____ _____		_____ _____	
_____ _____		_____ _____	
_____ _____		_____ _____	
_____ _____		TOTAL CALORIES/POINTS _____	

Calories/Points Tracker

DAILY GOAL _____

FRI

FOODS	CALORIES/POINTS	FOODS	CALORIES/POINTS
B_____	____	D_____	____
_____	____	_____	____
_____	____	_____	____
_____	____	_____	____
_____	____	_____	____
_____	____	_____	____
L_____	____	S_____	____
_____	____	_____	____
_____	____	_____	____
_____	____	_____	____
_____	____	_____	____
_____	____	TOTAL CALORIES/POINTS ____

SAT

FOODS	CALORIES/POINTS	FOODS	CALORIES/POINTS
B_____	____	D_____	____
_____	____	_____	____
_____	____	_____	____
_____	____	_____	____
_____	____	_____	____
_____	____	_____	____
L_____	____	S_____	____
_____	____	_____	____
_____	____	_____	____
_____	____	_____	____
_____	____	_____	____
_____	____	TOTAL CALORIES/POINTS ____

DATE _____ / __ / _____ TO _____ / __ / _____

SUN

FOODS	CALORIES/POINTS	FOODS	CALORIES/POINTS
B_____	____	D_____	____
_____	____	_____	____
_____	____	_____	____
_____	____	_____	____
_____	____	_____	____
L_____	____	S_____	____
_____	____	_____	____
_____	____	_____	____
_____	____	_____	____
_____	____		
_____	____	TOTAL CALORIES/POINTS ____	

Exercise Tracker

ACTIVITY	DISTANCE/DURATION/INTENSITY	CALORIES BURNED

Weekly Meal Planner

Weekly Goals _____

_____

_____

_____

_____

> "Nothing is impossible, the word itself says, 'I'm possible'!"
>
> **AUDREY HEPBURN**

MON

TUE

WED

THU

FRI

SAT

SUN

Calories/Points Tracker

MON

FOODS	CALORIES/POINTS
B_____	_____
_____	_____
_____	_____
_____	_____
_____	_____
L_____	_____
_____	_____
_____	_____
_____	_____
_____	_____

FOODS	CALORIES/POINTS
D_____	_____
_____	_____
_____	_____
_____	_____
_____	_____
S_____	_____
_____	_____
_____	_____
_____	_____
TOTAL CALORIES/POINTS	_____

TUE

FOODS	CALORIES/POINTS
B_____	_____
_____	_____
_____	_____
_____	_____
_____	_____
L_____	_____
_____	_____
_____	_____
_____	_____
_____	_____

FOODS	CALORIES/POINTS
D_____	_____
_____	_____
_____	_____
_____	_____
_____	_____
S_____	_____
_____	_____
_____	_____
_____	_____
TOTAL CALORIES/POINTS	_____

DATE ___ / ___ / ___ TO ___ / ___ / ___

FOODS	CALORIES/POINTS	FOODS	CALORIES/POINTS
B_____	_____	D_____	_____
_____	_____	_____	_____
_____	_____	_____	_____
_____	_____	_____	_____
_____	_____	_____	_____
_____	_____	_____	_____
L_____	_____	S_____	_____
_____	_____	_____	_____
_____	_____	_____	_____
_____	_____	_____	_____
_____	_____	_____	_____
_____	_____	TOTAL CALORIES/POINTS _____

FOODS	CALORIES/POINTS	FOODS	CALORIES/POINTS
B_____	_____	D_____	_____
_____	_____	_____	_____
_____	_____	_____	_____
_____	_____	_____	_____
_____	_____	_____	_____
_____	_____	_____	_____
L_____	_____	S_____	_____
_____	_____	_____	_____
_____	_____	_____	_____
_____	_____	_____	_____
_____	_____	_____	_____
_____	_____	TOTAL CALORIES/POINTS _____

Calories/Points Tracker

DAILY GOAL _____

	FOODS	CALORIES/POINTS	FOODS	CALORIES/POINTS

FRI

FOODS — CALORIES/POINTS

B _____ _____
_____ _____
_____ _____
_____ _____
_____ _____

L _____ _____
_____ _____
_____ _____
_____ _____
_____ _____

FOODS — CALORIES/POINTS

D _____ _____
_____ _____
_____ _____
_____ _____
_____ _____

S _____ _____
_____ _____
_____ _____
_____ _____

TOTAL CALORIES/POINTS _____

SAT

FOODS — CALORIES/POINTS

B _____ _____
_____ _____
_____ _____
_____ _____
_____ _____

L _____ _____
_____ _____
_____ _____
_____ _____
_____ _____

FOODS — CALORIES/POINTS

D _____ _____
_____ _____
_____ _____
_____ _____
_____ _____

S _____ _____
_____ _____
_____ _____
_____ _____

TOTAL CALORIES/POINTS _____

DATE ___ / ___ / ___ TO ___ / ___ / ___

FOODS	CALORIES/ POINTS	FOODS	CALORIES/ POINTS
B _____	_____	D _____	_____
_____	_____	_____	_____
_____	_____	_____	_____
_____	_____	_____	_____
_____	_____	_____	_____
_____	_____	_____	_____
L _____	_____	S _____	_____
_____	_____	_____	_____
_____	_____	_____	_____
_____	_____	_____	_____
_____	_____	TOTAL CALORIES/POINTS _____
_____	_____		

Exercise Tracker

ACTIVITY	DISTANCE/ DURATION/INTENSITY	CALORIES BURNED
_____	_____	_____
_____	_____	_____
_____	_____	_____
_____	_____	_____
_____	_____	_____
_____	_____	_____
_____	_____	_____
_____	_____	_____

Weekly Meal Planner

Weekly Goals _____

_____

_____

_____

_____

superfood

CHERRIES

Summer is the season for cherries. Snack on them plain, toss them into salads, or make a sauce with them for pork, which is delicious paired with fruit.

MON

TUE

WED

Calories/Points Tracker

MON

FOODS   CALORIES/ POINTS

B_____   _____
_____   _____
_____   _____
_____   _____
_____   _____

L_____   _____
_____   _____
_____   _____
_____   _____
_____   _____

FOODS   CALORIES/ POINTS

D_____   _____
_____   _____
_____   _____
_____   _____
_____   _____

S_____   _____
_____   _____
_____   _____
_____   _____

TOTAL CALORIES/POINTS _____

TUE

FOODS   CALORIES/ POINTS

B_____   _____
_____   _____
_____   _____
_____   _____
_____   _____

L_____   _____
_____   _____
_____   _____
_____   _____
_____   _____

FOODS   CALORIES/ POINTS

D_____   _____
_____   _____
_____   _____
_____   _____
_____   _____

S_____   _____
_____   _____
_____   _____
_____   _____

TOTAL CALORIES/POINTS _____

WED

FOODS	CALORIES/POINTS
B _____	____
_____	____
_____	____
_____	____
_____	____
_____	____
L _____	____
_____	____
_____	____
_____	____
_____	____
_____	____

FOODS	CALORIES/POINTS
D _____	____
_____	____
_____	____
_____	____
_____	____
_____	____
S _____	____
_____	____
_____	____
_____	____
TOTAL CALORIES/POINTS ____

THU

FOODS	CALORIES/POINTS
B _____	____
_____	____
_____	____
_____	____
_____	____
_____	____
L _____	____
_____	____
_____	____
_____	____
_____	____
_____	____

FOODS	CALORIES/POINTS
D _____	____
_____	____
_____	____
_____	____
_____	____
_____	____
S _____	____
_____	____
_____	____
_____	____
TOTAL CALORIES/POINTS ____

Calories/Points Tracker

DAILY GOAL _____

FRI

FOODS   CALORIES/ POINTS

B _____ _____

_____ _____

_____ _____

_____ _____

_____ _____

_____ _____

L _____ _____

_____ _____

_____ _____

_____ _____

_____ _____

_____ _____

FOODS   CALORIES/ POINTS

D _____ _____

_____ _____

_____ _____

_____ _____

_____ _____

S _____ _____

_____ _____

_____ _____

_____ _____

TOTAL CALORIES/POINTS _____

SAT

FOODS   CALORIES/ POINTS

B _____ _____

_____ _____

_____ _____

_____ _____

_____ _____

L _____ _____

_____ _____

_____ _____

_____ _____

_____ _____

_____ _____

FOODS   CALORIES/ POINTS

D _____ _____

_____ _____

_____ _____

_____ _____

_____ _____

_____ _____

S _____ _____

_____ _____

_____ _____

_____ _____

TOTAL CALORIES/POINTS _____

SUN

FOODS	CALORIES/ POINTS	FOODS	CALORIES/ POINTS
B_____	_____	D_____	_____
_____	_____	_____	_____
_____	_____	_____	_____
_____	_____	_____	_____
_____	_____	_____	_____
_____	_____	_____	_____
_____	_____		
L_____	_____	S_____	_____
_____	_____	_____	_____
_____	_____	_____	_____
_____	_____	_____	_____
_____	_____		
_____	_____	TOTAL CALORIES/POINTS _____
_____	_____		

--- Exercise Tracker ---

ACTIVITY	DISTANCE/ DURATION/INTENSITY	CALORIES BURNED
_____	_____	_____
_____	_____	_____
_____	_____	_____
_____	_____	_____
_____	_____	_____
_____	_____	_____
_____	_____	_____

Mushroom-Kale Lasagna Rolls

MAKES 10 ROLLS; SERVES 10

2½ cups marinara sauce

5 cups kale, stems removed, finely chopped

1 teaspoon olive oil

2 garlic cloves, chopped

¼ teaspoon plus a pinch of kosher salt

Freshly ground black pepper

8 ounces mushrooms, finely chopped

15 ounces part-skim ricotta cheese (I like Polly-o)

½ cup grated Parmesan cheese

1 large egg, beaten

10 lasagna noodles, cooked (9 ounces dry)

3 ounces part-skim mozzarella cheese, shredded (10 tablespoons)

SERVING SIZE	1 roll
CALORIES	260.5
FAT	9 g
CHOLESTEROL	41 mg
CARBOHYDRATE	30 g
FIBER	3 g
PROTEIN	12 g
SUGAR	3.5 g
SODIUM	200 mg

Preheat the oven to 350°F.

Ladle about 1 cup of sauce on the bottom of a 9 x 12-inch baking dish.

Place the kale in a food processor and pulse a few times until chopped.

In a large saucepan set over medium heat, heat the oil. Add the garlic and cook, stirring, until golden, about 1 minute. Add the kale, ¼ teaspoon of the salt, and season with pepper; cook, stirring, about 5 minutes. Add the mushrooms and cook until soft, 5 to 6 minutes. Season with a pinch of salt and pepper. Transfer the mixture to a medium bowl and add the ricotta, Parmesan cheese, and egg.

Place a piece of wax paper on a work surface and lay the cooked lasagna noodles on it. Make sure the noodles are dry. Take ⅓ cup of the kale mixture and spread it evenly over a noodle. Roll it up carefully and place it into the baking dish seam side down. Repeat with the remaining noodles. Ladle 1 cup of sauce over the noodles in the baking dish and top each roll with 1 tablespoon mozzarella cheese. Cover the dish with foil.

Bake until the cheese melts, 40 minutes. Serve with extra sauce on the side.

Weekly Meal Planner

Weekly Goals _____

_____

_____

_____

_____

> "We are what we repeatedly do."
>
> ARISTOTLE

MON

_____

_____

_____

_____

TUE

_____

_____

_____

_____

WED

_____

_____

_____

THU

FRI

SAT

SUN

Calories/Points Tracker

DAILY GOAL _____

MON

FOODS	CALORIES/ POINTS	FOODS	CALORIES/ POINTS
B_____	_____	D_____	_____
_____	_____	_____	_____
_____	_____	_____	_____
_____	_____	_____	_____
_____	_____	_____	_____
_____	_____	_____	_____
L_____	_____	S_____	_____
_____	_____	_____	_____
_____	_____	_____	_____
_____	_____	_____	_____
_____	_____	_____	_____
_____	_____		
		TOTAL CALORIES/POINTS _____	

TUE

FOODS	CALORIES/ POINTS	FOODS	CALORIES/ POINTS
B_____	_____	D_____	_____
_____	_____	_____	_____
_____	_____	_____	_____
_____	_____	_____	_____
_____	_____	_____	_____
_____	_____	_____	_____
L_____	_____	S_____	_____
_____	_____	_____	_____
_____	_____	_____	_____
_____	_____	_____	_____
_____	_____	_____	_____
_____	_____		
		TOTAL CALORIES/POINTS _____	

WED

FOODS	CALORIES/ POINTS
B_____	_____
_____	_____
_____	_____
_____	_____
_____	_____
_____	_____
L_____	_____
_____	_____
_____	_____
_____	_____
_____	_____
_____	_____

FOODS	CALORIES/ POINTS
D_____	_____
_____	_____
_____	_____
_____	_____
_____	_____
_____	_____
_____	_____
S_____	_____
_____	_____
_____	_____
_____	_____
TOTAL CALORIES/POINTS	_____

THU

FOODS	CALORIES/ POINTS
B_____	_____
_____	_____
_____	_____
_____	_____
_____	_____
_____	_____
L_____	_____
_____	_____
_____	_____
_____	_____
_____	_____
_____	_____

FOODS	CALORIES/ POINTS
D_____	_____
_____	_____
_____	_____
_____	_____
_____	_____
_____	_____
_____	_____
S_____	_____
_____	_____
_____	_____
_____	_____
TOTAL CALORIES/POINTS	_____

Calories/Points Tracker

DAILY GOAL _____

FRI

FOODS	CALORIES/POINTS	FOODS	CALORIES/POINTS
B _____	_____	D _____	_____
_____	_____	_____	_____
_____	_____	_____	_____
_____	_____	_____	_____
_____	_____	_____	_____
_____	_____	_____	_____
L _____	_____	S _____	_____
_____	_____	_____	_____
_____	_____	_____	_____
_____	_____	_____	_____
_____	_____		
_____	_____	TOTAL CALORIES/POINTS _____	

SAT

FOODS	CALORIES/POINTS	FOODS	CALORIES/POINTS
B _____	_____	D _____	_____
_____	_____	_____	_____
_____	_____	_____	_____
_____	_____	_____	_____
_____	_____	_____	_____
_____	_____	_____	_____
L _____	_____	S _____	_____
_____	_____	_____	_____
_____	_____	_____	_____
_____	_____	_____	_____
_____	_____		
_____	_____	TOTAL CALORIES/POINTS _____	

DATE ___ / ___ / ___ TO ___ / ___ / ___

FOODS	CALORIES/ POINTS	FOODS	CALORIES/ POINTS
B_____	_____	D_____	_____
_____	_____	_____	_____
_____	_____	_____	_____
_____	_____	_____	_____
_____	_____	_____	_____
_____	_____	_____	_____
L_____	_____	S_____	_____
_____	_____	_____	_____
_____	_____	_____	_____
_____	_____	_____	_____
_____	_____	TOTAL CALORIES/POINTS _____

—————————— Exercise Tracker ——————————

ACTIVITY	DISTANCE/ DURATION/INTENSITY	CALORIES BURNED
_____	_____	_____
_____	_____	_____
_____	_____	_____
_____	_____	_____
_____	_____	_____
_____	_____	_____
_____	_____	_____

Weekly Meal Planner

Weekly Goals _____

_____

_____

_____

_____

> "Keep your face always toward the sunshine—and shadows will fall behind you."
>
> **WALT WHITMAN**

MON

_____

_____

_____

_____

TUE

_____

_____

_____

_____

WED

_____

_____

_____

_____

Calories/Points Tracker

MON

FOODS	CALORIES/POINTS	FOODS	CALORIES/POINTS
B_____	____	D_____	____
_____	____	_____	____
_____	____	_____	____
_____	____	_____	____
_____	____	_____	____
_____	____	_____	____
L_____	____	S_____	____
_____	____	_____	____
_____	____	_____	____
_____	____	_____	____
_____	____		
_____	____	TOTAL CALORIES/POINTS ____	

TUE

FOODS	CALORIES/POINTS	FOODS	CALORIES/POINTS
B_____	____	D_____	____
_____	____	_____	____
_____	____	_____	____
_____	____	_____	____
_____	____	_____	____
_____	____	_____	____
L_____	____	S_____	____
_____	____	_____	____
_____	____	_____	____
_____	____	_____	____
_____	____		
_____	____	TOTAL CALORIES/POINTS ____	

DATE _____ / _____ / _____ TO _____ / _____ / _____

FOODS	CALORIES/ POINTS	FOODS	CALORIES/ POINTS
B_____ _____		D_____ _____	
_____ _____		_____ _____	
_____ _____		_____ _____	
_____ _____		_____ _____	
_____ _____		_____ _____	
_____ _____		_____ _____	
L_____ _____		S_____ _____	
_____ _____		_____ _____	
_____ _____		_____ _____	
_____ _____		_____ _____	
_____ _____		_____ _____	
_____ _____		TOTAL CALORIES/POINTS _____	

FOODS	CALORIES/ POINTS	FOODS	CALORIES/ POINTS
B_____ _____		D_____ _____	
_____ _____		_____ _____	
_____ _____		_____ _____	
_____ _____		_____ _____	
_____ _____		_____ _____	
_____ _____		_____ _____	
L_____ _____		S_____ _____	
_____ _____		_____ _____	
_____ _____		_____ _____	
_____ _____		_____ _____	
_____ _____		_____ _____	
_____ _____		TOTAL CALORIES/POINTS _____	

Calories/Points Tracker

FOODS CALORIES/ POINTS

FOODS CALORIES/ POINTS

FRI

B _____ _____
_____ _____
_____ _____
_____ _____
_____ _____
_____ _____

L _____ _____
_____ _____
_____ _____
_____ _____
_____ _____

D _____ _____
_____ _____
_____ _____
_____ _____
_____ _____
_____ _____

S _____ _____
_____ _____
_____ _____
_____ _____

TOTAL CALORIES/POINTS _____

FOODS CALORIES/ POINTS

FOODS CALORIES/ POINTS

SAT

B _____ _____
_____ _____
_____ _____
_____ _____
_____ _____

L _____ _____
_____ _____
_____ _____
_____ _____
_____ _____

D _____ _____
_____ _____
_____ _____
_____ _____
_____ _____

S _____ _____
_____ _____
_____ _____
_____ _____

TOTAL CALORIES/POINTS _____

SUN

FOODS	CALORIES/ POINTS	FOODS	CALORIES/ POINTS
B_____ ___		D_____ ___	
_____ ___		_____ ___	
_____ ___		_____ ___	
_____ ___		_____ ___	
_____ ___		_____ ___	
_____ ___		_____ ___	
L_____ ___		S_____ ___	
_____ ___		_____ ___	
_____ ___		_____ ___	
_____ ___		_____ ___	
_____ ___			
_____ ___		TOTAL CALORIES/POINTS ___	

—————— Exercise Tracker ——————

ACTIVITY	DISTANCE/ DURATION/INTENSITY	CALORIES BURNED
_____	_____	_____
_____	_____	_____
_____	_____	_____
_____	_____	_____
_____	_____	_____
_____	_____	_____
_____	_____	_____
_____	_____	_____

Weekly Meal Planner

Weekly Goals _____

_____

_____

_____

_____

superfood

SWEET POTATOES

Trust me when I say that roasting
sweet potatoes is the way to go!
Microwaving will get them cooked, but
the caramelization that comes through
roasting is worth the extra time.

MON

TUE

WED

Calories/Points Tracker

DAILY GOAL

MON

FOODS CALORIES/POINTS

B_____ _____
_____ _____
_____ _____
_____ _____
_____ _____
_____ _____

L_____ _____
_____ _____
_____ _____
_____ _____
_____ _____
_____ _____

FOODS CALORIES/POINTS

D_____ _____
_____ _____
_____ _____
_____ _____
_____ _____
_____ _____

S_____ _____
_____ _____
_____ _____
_____ _____

TOTAL CALORIES/POINTS _____

TUE

FOODS CALORIES/POINTS

B_____ _____
_____ _____
_____ _____
_____ _____
_____ _____
_____ _____

L_____ _____
_____ _____
_____ _____
_____ _____
_____ _____
_____ _____

FOODS CALORIES/POINTS

D_____ _____
_____ _____
_____ _____
_____ _____
_____ _____
_____ _____

S_____ _____
_____ _____
_____ _____
_____ _____

TOTAL CALORIES/POINTS _____

DATE _____ / _____ / _____ TO _____ / _____ / _____

FOODS	CALORIES/ POINTS	FOODS	CALORIES/ POINTS
B_____ ____		D_____ ____	
_____ ____		_____ ____	
_____ ____		_____ ____	
_____ ____		_____ ____	
_____ ____		_____ ____	
_____ ____		_____ ____	
L_____ ____		S_____ ____	
_____ ____		_____ ____	
_____ ____		_____ ____	
_____ ____		_____ ____	
_____ ____		TOTAL CALORIES/POINTS ____	

FOODS	CALORIES/ POINTS	FOODS	CALORIES/ POINTS
B_____ ____		D_____ ____	
_____ ____		_____ ____	
_____ ____		_____ ____	
_____ ____		_____ ____	
_____ ____		_____ ____	
_____ ____		_____ ____	
L_____ ____		S_____ ____	
_____ ____		_____ ____	
_____ ____		_____ ____	
_____ ____		_____ ____	
_____ ____		TOTAL CALORIES/POINTS ____	

Calories/Points Tracker

DAILY GOAL _____

FRI

FOODS	CALORIES/ POINTS		FOODS	CALORIES/ POINTS
B_____	_____		D_____	_____
_____	_____		_____	_____
_____	_____		_____	_____
_____	_____		_____	_____
_____	_____		_____	_____
_____	_____		_____	_____
L_____	_____		S_____	_____
_____	_____		_____	_____
_____	_____		_____	_____
_____	_____		_____	_____
_____	_____			
_____	_____		TOTAL CALORIES/POINTS _____	

SAT

FOODS	CALORIES/ POINTS		FOODS	CALORIES/ POINTS
B_____	_____		D_____	_____
_____	_____		_____	_____
_____	_____		_____	_____
_____	_____		_____	_____
_____	_____		_____	_____
_____	_____		_____	_____
L_____	_____		S_____	_____
_____	_____		_____	_____
_____	_____		_____	_____
_____	_____		_____	_____
_____	_____			
_____	_____		TOTAL CALORIES/POINTS _____	

DATE ___ / ___ / ___ TO ___ / ___ / ___

FOODS	CALORIES/POINTS	FOODS	CALORIES/POINTS
B_____	____	D_____	____
_____	____	_____	____
_____	____	_____	____
_____	____	_____	____
_____	____	_____	____
_____	____	_____	____
L_____	____	S_____	____
_____	____	_____	____
_____	____	_____	____
_____	____	_____	____
_____	____		
_____	____	TOTAL CALORIES/POINTS ____	

——————————— Exercise Tracker ———————————

ACTIVITY	DISTANCE/DURATION/INTENSITY	CALORIES BURNED
_____	_____	_____
_____	_____	_____
_____	_____	_____
_____	_____	_____
_____	_____	_____
_____	_____	_____
_____	_____	_____
_____	_____	_____

Sweet Potato Irish Nachos

SERVES 4

FOR THE POTATOES

Nonstick cooking spray

4 medium sweet potatoes
(about 7 ounces each)

1 tablespoon olive oil

1½ teaspoons paprika

1 teaspoon garlic powder

Pinch of cayenne pepper

1 teaspoon kosher salt

Freshly ground black pepper

FOR THE TOPPING

½ red bell pepper, thinly sliced

⅓ cup grated sharp shredded
cheddar cheese
(I like Cabot)

½ cup light pepper Jack cheese

1 medium scallion, chopped

4 tablespoons diced fresh
tomato

1 tablespoon chopped fresh
cilantro

Pickled jalapeño slices (optional)

Sliced black olives (optional)

Salsa, for dipping (optional)

SERVING SIZE	1 sweet potato with toppings
CALORIES	332
FAT	9.5 g
CHOLESTEROL	10 mg
CARBOHYDRATE	52 g
FIBER	7 g
PROTEIN	9.5 g
SUGAR	0 g
SODIUM	453 mg

Preheat the oven to 425°F. Lightly spray a baking sheet with nonstick cooking spray.

Cut each sweet potato in half, and then cut each half into 3 equal wedges to make 24 wedges total. Put the wedges in a large bowl, add the oil, and toss well. Add the paprika, garlic powder, cayenne, and salt, and season with pepper. Toss to coat. Arrange wedges in a single layer on the prepared baking sheet.

Bake until browned, flipping halfway, 18 to 20 minutes. Remove from the oven and transfer the wedges to four small oven-safe dishes (or one large dish for sharing).

Top the wedges with the bell peppers and cheddar and Jack cheeses and return to the oven until the cheese melts, about 2 minutes. Remove from the oven and scatter with the scallions, tomato, and cilantro, and the jalapeño and black olives, if using. Serve with salsa on the side, if desired.

Weekly Meal Planner

Weekly Goals _____

_____

_____

_____

_____

> "Whatever the mind of man can conceive and believe, it can achieve."
>
> — NAPOLEON HILL

MON

TUE

WED

DATE ___/___/___ TO ___/___/___

THU

FRI

SAT

SUN

Calories/Points Tracker

MON

FOODS	CALORIES/POINTS
B_____	_____
_____	_____
_____	_____
_____	_____
_____	_____
_____	_____
L_____	_____
_____	_____
_____	_____
_____	_____
_____	_____

FOODS	CALORIES/POINTS
D_____	_____
_____	_____
_____	_____
_____	_____
_____	_____
_____	_____
S_____	_____
_____	_____
_____	_____
_____	_____
TOTAL CALORIES/POINTS	_____

TUE

FOODS	CALORIES/POINTS
B_____	_____
_____	_____
_____	_____
_____	_____
_____	_____
_____	_____
L_____	_____
_____	_____
_____	_____
_____	_____
_____	_____

FOODS	CALORIES/POINTS
D_____	_____
_____	_____
_____	_____
_____	_____
_____	_____
_____	_____
S_____	_____
_____	_____
_____	_____
_____	_____
TOTAL CALORIES/POINTS	_____

DATE _____ / _____ / _____ TO _____ / _____ / _____

FOODS	CALORIES/ POINTS	FOODS	CALORIES/ POINTS
B _____	_____	D _____	_____
_____	_____	_____	_____
_____	_____	_____	_____
_____	_____	_____	_____
_____	_____	_____	_____
_____	_____	_____	_____
L _____	_____	S _____	_____
_____	_____	_____	_____
_____	_____	_____	_____
_____	_____	_____	_____
_____	_____		
_____	_____	TOTAL CALORIES/POINTS _____	

FOODS	CALORIES/ POINTS	FOODS	CALORIES/ POINTS
B _____	_____	D _____	_____
_____	_____	_____	_____
_____	_____	_____	_____
_____	_____	_____	_____
_____	_____	_____	_____
_____	_____	_____	_____
L _____	_____	S _____	_____
_____	_____	_____	_____
_____	_____	_____	_____
_____	_____	_____	_____
_____	_____		
_____	_____	TOTAL CALORIES/POINTS _____	

Calories/Points Tracker

DAILY GOAL

FOODS	CALORIES/POINTS	FOODS	CALORIES/POINTS

FRI

B _____ _____

_____ _____

_____ _____

_____ _____

_____ _____

_____ _____

L _____ _____

_____ _____

_____ _____

_____ _____

_____ _____

D _____ _____

_____ _____

_____ _____

_____ _____

_____ _____

_____ _____

S _____ _____

_____ _____

_____ _____

_____ _____

TOTAL CALORIES/POINTS _____

FOODS	CALORIES/POINTS	FOODS	CALORIES/POINTS

SAT

B _____ _____

_____ _____

_____ _____

_____ _____

_____ _____

_____ _____

L _____ _____

_____ _____

_____ _____

_____ _____

_____ _____

D _____ _____

_____ _____

_____ _____

_____ _____

_____ _____

_____ _____

S _____ _____

_____ _____

_____ _____

_____ _____

TOTAL CALORIES/POINTS _____

DATE ___ / ___ / ___ TO ___ / ___ / ___

FOODS	CALORIES/POINTS	FOODS	CALORIES/POINTS
B_____	_____	D_____	_____
_____	_____	_____	_____
_____	_____	_____	_____
_____	_____	_____	_____
_____	_____	_____	_____
_____	_____	_____	_____
L_____	_____	S_____	_____
_____	_____	_____	_____
_____	_____	_____	_____
_____	_____	_____	_____
_____	_____		
_____	_____	TOTAL CALORIES/POINTS _____	

Exercise Tracker

ACTIVITY	DISTANCE/DURATION/INTENSITY	CALORIES BURNED
_____	_____	_____
_____	_____	_____
_____	_____	_____
_____	_____	_____
_____	_____	_____
_____	_____	_____
_____	_____	_____
_____	_____	_____

Weekly Meal Planner

Weekly Goals _____

_____

_____

_____

_____

superfood

BLUEBERRIES

Try tossing small but powerful blueberries in yogurt, cereal, or a smoothie,
or just eat a handful on the go.

MON

TUE

WED

Calories/Points Tracker

DAILY GOAL _____

MON

FOODS	CALORIES/ POINTS	FOODS	CALORIES/ POINTS
B_____	____	D_____	____
_____	____	_____	____
_____	____	_____	____
_____	____	_____	____
_____	____	_____	____
_____	____	_____	____
L_____	____	S_____	____
_____	____	_____	____
_____	____	_____	____
_____	____	_____	____
_____	____		
_____	____	TOTAL CALORIES/POINTS ____	

TUE

FOODS	CALORIES/ POINTS	FOODS	CALORIES/ POINTS
B_____	____	D_____	____
_____	____	_____	____
_____	____	_____	____
_____	____	_____	____
_____	____	_____	____
_____	____	_____	____
L_____	____	S_____	____
_____	____	_____	____
_____	____	_____	____
_____	____	_____	____
_____	____		
_____	____	TOTAL CALORIES/POINTS ____	

DATE _____ / _____ / _____ TO _____ / _____ / _____

FOODS	CALORIES/ POINTS	FOODS	CALORIES/ POINTS
B		D	
L		S	
		TOTAL CALORIES/POINTS _____	

FOODS	CALORIES/ POINTS	FOODS	CALORIES/ POINTS
B		D	
L		S	
		TOTAL CALORIES/POINTS _____	

Calories/Points Tracker

DAILY GOAL _____

FRI

FOODS	CALORIES/ POINTS	FOODS	CALORIES/ POINTS
B_____	____	D_____	____
_____	____	_____	____
_____	____	_____	____
_____	____	_____	____
_____	____	_____	____
_____	____		
L_____	____	S_____	____
_____	____	_____	____
_____	____	_____	____
_____	____	_____	____
_____	____	_____	____
_____	____	TOTAL CALORIES/POINTS ____	

SAT

FOODS	CALORIES/ POINTS	FOODS	CALORIES/ POINTS
B_____	____	D_____	____
_____	____	_____	____
_____	____	_____	____
_____	____	_____	____
_____	____	_____	____
_____	____		
L_____	____	S_____	____
_____	____	_____	____
_____	____	_____	____
_____	____	_____	____
_____	____	_____	____
_____	____	TOTAL CALORIES/POINTS ____	

DATE ___ / ___ / ___ TO ___ / ___ / ___

FOODS	CALORIES/ POINTS	FOODS	CALORIES/ POINTS
B _____	_____	D _____	_____
_____	_____	_____	_____
_____	_____	_____	_____
_____	_____	_____	_____
_____	_____	_____	_____
_____	_____	_____	_____
L _____	_____	S _____	_____
_____	_____	_____	_____
_____	_____	_____	_____
_____	_____	_____	_____
_____	_____		
_____	_____	TOTAL CALORIES/POINTS _____	

Exercise Tracker

ACTIVITY	DISTANCE/ DURATION/INTENSITY	CALORIES BURNED
_____	_____	_____
_____	_____	_____
_____	_____	_____
_____	_____	_____
_____	_____	_____
_____	_____	_____
_____	_____	_____
_____	_____	_____

Weekly Meal Planner

Weekly Goals _____

_____

_____

_____

_____

> "The most difficult thing is the decision to act, the rest is merely tenacity."
>
> **AMELIA EARHART**

MON

TUE

WED

Calories/Points Tracker

DAILY GOAL _____

MON

FOODS	CALORIES/POINTS	FOODS	CALORIES/POINTS
B_____	_____	D_____	_____
_____	_____	_____	_____
_____	_____	_____	_____
_____	_____	_____	_____
_____	_____	_____	_____
_____	_____	_____	_____
L_____	_____	S_____	_____
_____	_____	_____	_____
_____	_____	_____	_____
_____	_____	_____	_____
_____	_____		
_____	_____	TOTAL CALORIES/POINTS	_____

TUE

FOODS	CALORIES/POINTS	FOODS	CALORIES/POINTS
B_____	_____	D_____	_____
_____	_____	_____	_____
_____	_____	_____	_____
_____	_____	_____	_____
_____	_____	_____	_____
_____	_____	_____	_____
L_____	_____	S_____	_____
_____	_____	_____	_____
_____	_____	_____	_____
_____	_____	_____	_____
_____	_____		
_____	_____	TOTAL CALORIES/POINTS	_____

FOODS	CALORIES/POINTS	FOODS	CALORIES/POINTS
B_____	_____	D_____	_____
_____	_____	_____	_____
_____	_____	_____	_____
_____	_____	_____	_____
_____	_____	_____	_____
_____	_____	_____	_____
L_____	_____	S_____	_____
_____	_____	_____	_____
_____	_____	_____	_____
_____	_____	_____	_____
_____	_____	TOTAL CALORIES/POINTS	_____

FOODS	CALORIES/POINTS	FOODS	CALORIES/POINTS
B_____	_____	D_____	_____
_____	_____	_____	_____
_____	_____	_____	_____
_____	_____	_____	_____
_____	_____	_____	_____
_____	_____	_____	_____
L_____	_____	S_____	_____
_____	_____	_____	_____
_____	_____	_____	_____
_____	_____	_____	_____
_____	_____	TOTAL CALORIES/POINTS	_____

Calories/Points Tracker

DAILY GOAL _____

FRI

FOODS	CALORIES/POINTS	FOODS	CALORIES/POINTS
B_____ _____		D_____ _____	
_____ _____		_____ _____	
_____ _____		_____ _____	
_____ _____		_____ _____	
_____ _____		_____ _____	
_____ _____		_____ _____	
L_____ _____		S_____ _____	
_____ _____		_____ _____	
_____ _____		_____ _____	
_____ _____		_____ _____	
_____ _____			
_____ _____		TOTAL CALORIES/POINTS _____	

SAT

FOODS	CALORIES/POINTS	FOODS	CALORIES/POINTS
B_____ _____		D_____ _____	
_____ _____		_____ _____	
_____ _____		_____ _____	
_____ _____		_____ _____	
_____ _____		_____ _____	
_____ _____		_____ _____	
L_____ _____		S_____ _____	
_____ _____		_____ _____	
_____ _____		_____ _____	
_____ _____		_____ _____	
_____ _____			
_____ _____		TOTAL CALORIES/POINTS _____	

DATE ___/___/___ TO ___/___/___

FOODS	CALORIES/ POINTS	FOODS	CALORIES/ POINTS
B_____ ____		D_____ ____	
_____ ____		_____ ____	
_____ ____		_____ ____	
_____ ____		_____ ____	
_____ ____		_____ ____	
_____ ____		_____ ____	
L_____ ____		S_____ ____	
_____ ____		_____ ____	
_____ ____		_____ ____	
_____ ____		_____ ____	
_____ ____			
_____ ____		TOTAL CALORIES/POINTS ____	

―――――――――― Exercise Tracker ――――――――――

ACTIVITY	DISTANCE/ DURATION/INTENSITY	CALORIES BURNED
_____	_____	_____
_____	_____	_____
_____	_____	_____
_____	_____	_____
_____	_____	_____
_____	_____	_____
_____	_____	_____
_____	_____	_____

Broccoli-and-Cheese Mini Egg Omelets

MAKES 9 MINI OMELETS; SERVES 4½

Nonstick cooking spray

4 cups broccoli florets

1 teaspoon olive oil

¼ teaspoon plus a pinch of kosher salt

Freshly ground black pepper

4 large eggs

1 cup egg whites

¼ cup reduced-fat shredded cheddar cheese

¼ cup grated Pecorino Romano cheese

SERVING SIZE	2 omelets
CALORIES	155
FAT	7.5 g
CHOLESTEROL	170 mg
CARBOHYDRATE	5 g
FIBER	2.5 g
PROTEIN	16.5 g
SUGAR	0 g
SODIUM	348.5 mg

Preheat the oven to 350°F. Spray nine cups of a standard nonstick muffin tin with nonstick cooking spray.

Steam the broccoli in a little boiling water until tender, 6 to 7 minutes. Chop the broccoli, transfer to a bowl, add the olive oil and ¼ teaspoon of the salt, and season with pepper. Mix well. Spoon the mixture evenly into nine of the cups in the prepared tin.

In a medium bowl, beat the eggs, egg whites, and cheddar cheese, and season with a pinch of salt and pepper. Pour the mixture over the broccoli in the tin until the cups are a little more than three-fourths full. Top with the Pecorino Romano cheese.

Bake until cooked through, about 20 minutes. Serve immediately. Wrap any leftovers in plastic wrap and store in the refrigerator to enjoy during the week.

Weekly Meal Planner

Weekly Goals —————————

—————————————————

—————————————————

—————————————————

—————————————————

MON

TUE

WED

Calories/Points Tracker

DAILY GOAL

MON

FOODS	CALORIES/POINTS	FOODS	CALORIES/POINTS
B_____	_____	D_____	_____
_____	_____	_____	_____
_____	_____	_____	_____
_____	_____	_____	_____
_____	_____	_____	_____
_____	_____	_____	_____
L_____	_____	S_____	_____
_____	_____	_____	_____
_____	_____	_____	_____
_____	_____	_____	_____
_____	_____		
_____	_____	TOTAL CALORIES/POINTS _____	

TUE

FOODS	CALORIES/POINTS	FOODS	CALORIES/POINTS
B_____	_____	D_____	_____
_____	_____	_____	_____
_____	_____	_____	_____
_____	_____	_____	_____
_____	_____	_____	_____
_____	_____	_____	_____
L_____	_____	S_____	_____
_____	_____	_____	_____
_____	_____	_____	_____
_____	_____	_____	_____
_____	_____		
_____	_____	TOTAL CALORIES/POINTS _____	

DATE ___/___/___ TO ___/___/___

FOODS	CALORIES/POINTS	FOODS	CALORIES/POINTS
B _____	____	D _____	____
_____	____	_____	____
_____	____	_____	____
_____	____	_____	____
_____	____	_____	____
_____	____	_____	____
L _____	____	S _____	____
_____	____	_____	____
_____	____	_____	____
_____	____	_____	____
_____	____	TOTAL CALORIES/POINTS ____
_____	____		

FOODS	CALORIES/POINTS	FOODS	CALORIES/POINTS
B _____	____	D _____	____
_____	____	_____	____
_____	____	_____	____
_____	____	_____	____
_____	____	_____	____
_____	____	_____	____
L _____	____	S _____	____
_____	____	_____	____
_____	____	_____	____
_____	____	_____	____
_____	____	TOTAL CALORIES/POINTS ____
_____	____		

Calories/Points Tracker

FRI

FOODS	CALORIES/POINTS	FOODS	CALORIES/POINTS
B _____	_____	D _____	_____
_____	_____	_____	_____
_____	_____	_____	_____
_____	_____	_____	_____
_____	_____	_____	_____
_____	_____	_____	_____
L _____	_____	S _____	_____
_____	_____	_____	_____
_____	_____	_____	_____
_____	_____	_____	_____
_____	_____	_____	_____
_____	_____	TOTAL CALORIES/POINTS _____	

SAT

FOODS	CALORIES/POINTS	FOODS	CALORIES/POINTS
B _____	_____	D _____	_____
_____	_____	_____	_____
_____	_____	_____	_____
_____	_____	_____	_____
_____	_____	_____	_____
_____	_____	_____	_____
L _____	_____	S _____	_____
_____	_____	_____	_____
_____	_____	_____	_____
_____	_____	_____	_____
_____	_____	_____	_____
_____	_____	TOTAL CALORIES/POINTS _____	

SUN

DATE ___ / ___ / ___ TO ___ / ___ / ___

FOODS	CALORIES/POINTS	FOODS	CALORIES/POINTS
B_____	_____	D_____	_____
_____	_____	_____	_____
_____	_____	_____	_____
_____	_____	_____	_____
_____	_____	_____	_____
_____	_____	_____	_____
L_____	_____	S_____	_____
_____	_____	_____	_____
_____	_____	_____	_____
_____	_____	_____	_____
_____	_____		
_____	_____	TOTAL CALORIES/POINTS _____	

——————— Exercise Tracker ———————

ACTIVITY	DISTANCE/DURATION/INTENSITY	CALORIES BURNED
_____	_____	_____
_____	_____	_____
_____	_____	_____
_____	_____	_____
_____	_____	_____
_____	_____	_____
_____	_____	_____
_____	_____	_____

Weekly Meal Planner

Weekly Goals _____

_____

_____

_____

_____

superfood

WALNUTS

I love to toast walnuts to add to salads. Just put them on a baking sheet in a 350°F oven, stirring halfway through, until golden brown, about 10 minutes— and you're set!

MON

TUE

WED

Calories/Points Tracker

MON

FOODS	CALORIES/ POINTS	FOODS	CALORIES/ POINTS
B_____	_____	D_____	_____
_____	_____	_____	_____
_____	_____	_____	_____
_____	_____	_____	_____
_____	_____	_____	_____
L_____	_____	S_____	_____
_____	_____	_____	_____
_____	_____	_____	_____
_____	_____	_____	_____
_____	_____	TOTAL CALORIES/POINTS _____	

TUE

FOODS	CALORIES/ POINTS	FOODS	CALORIES/ POINTS
B_____	_____	D_____	_____
_____	_____	_____	_____
_____	_____	_____	_____
_____	_____	_____	_____
_____	_____	_____	_____
L_____	_____	S_____	_____
_____	_____	_____	_____
_____	_____	_____	_____
_____	_____	_____	_____
_____	_____	TOTAL CALORIES/POINTS _____	

FOODS	CALORIES/POINTS	FOODS	CALORIES/POINTS
B_____	_____	D_____	_____
_____	_____	_____	_____
_____	_____	_____	_____
_____	_____	_____	_____
_____	_____	_____	_____
_____	_____	_____	_____
L_____	_____	S_____	_____
_____	_____	_____	_____
_____	_____	_____	_____
_____	_____	_____	_____
_____	_____	_____	_____
_____	_____	TOTAL CALORIES/POINTS _____	

FOODS	CALORIES/POINTS	FOODS	CALORIES/POINTS
B_____	_____	D_____	_____
_____	_____	_____	_____
_____	_____	_____	_____
_____	_____	_____	_____
_____	_____	_____	_____
_____	_____	_____	_____
L_____	_____	S_____	_____
_____	_____	_____	_____
_____	_____	_____	_____
_____	_____	_____	_____
_____	_____	_____	_____
_____	_____	TOTAL CALORIES/POINTS _____	

Calories/Points Tracker

FRI

FOODS   CALORIES/ POINTS

B_____ _____

_____ _____

_____ _____

_____ _____

_____ _____

_____ _____

L_____ _____

_____ _____

_____ _____

_____ _____

_____ _____

_____ _____

FOODS   CALORIES/ POINTS

D_____ _____

_____ _____

_____ _____

_____ _____

_____ _____

_____ _____

S_____ _____

_____ _____

_____ _____

_____ _____

TOTAL CALORIES/POINTS _____

SAT

FOODS   CALORIES/ POINTS

B_____ _____

_____ _____

_____ _____

_____ _____

_____ _____

_____ _____

L_____ _____

_____ _____

_____ _____

_____ _____

_____ _____

_____ _____

FOODS   CALORIES/ POINTS

D_____ _____

_____ _____

_____ _____

_____ _____

_____ _____

_____ _____

S_____ _____

_____ _____

_____ _____

_____ _____

TOTAL CALORIES/POINTS _____

DATE ___ / ___ / ___ TO ___ / ___ / ___

FOODS	CALORIES/ POINTS	FOODS	CALORIES/ POINTS
B_____	_____	D_____	_____
_____	_____	_____	_____
_____	_____	_____	_____
_____	_____	_____	_____
_____	_____	_____	_____
_____	_____	_____	_____
L_____	_____	S_____	_____
_____	_____	_____	_____
_____	_____	_____	_____
_____	_____	_____	_____
_____	_____		
_____	_____	TOTAL CALORIES/POINTS _____	

Exercise Tracker

ACTIVITY	DISTANCE/ DURATION/INTENSITY	CALORIES BURNED
_____	_____	_____
_____	_____	_____
_____	_____	_____
_____	_____	_____
_____	_____	_____
_____	_____	_____
_____	_____	_____
_____	_____	_____

Weekly Meal Planner

Weekly Goals _____

_____

_____

_____

_____

> "You can never cross the ocean until you have the courage to lose sight of the shore."
>
> CHRISTOPHER COLUMBUS

MON

TUE

WED

THU

FRI

SAT

SUN

Calories/Points Tracker

DAILY GOAL

MON

FOODS	CALORIES/POINTS	FOODS	CALORIES/POINTS
B _____	_____	D _____	_____
_____	_____	_____	_____
_____	_____	_____	_____
_____	_____	_____	_____
_____	_____	_____	_____
L _____	_____	S _____	_____
_____	_____	_____	_____
_____	_____	_____	_____
_____	_____	_____	_____
_____	_____	TOTAL CALORIES/POINTS _____	

TUE

FOODS	CALORIES/POINTS	FOODS	CALORIES/POINTS
B _____	_____	D _____	_____
_____	_____	_____	_____
_____	_____	_____	_____
_____	_____	_____	_____
_____	_____	_____	_____
L _____	_____	S _____	_____
_____	_____	_____	_____
_____	_____	_____	_____
_____	_____	_____	_____
_____	_____	TOTAL CALORIES/POINTS _____	

DATE _____ / _____ / _____ TO _____ / _____ / _____

FOODS	CALORIES/ POINTS	FOODS	CALORIES/ POINTS
B _____ _____		D _____ _____	
_____ _____		_____ _____	
_____ _____		_____ _____	
_____ _____		_____ _____	
_____ _____		_____ _____	
_____ _____		_____ _____	
L _____ _____		S _____ _____	
_____ _____		_____ _____	
_____ _____		_____ _____	
_____ _____		_____ _____	
_____ _____		TOTAL CALORIES/POINTS _____	

FOODS	CALORIES/ POINTS	FOODS	CALORIES/ POINTS
B _____ _____		D _____ _____	
_____ _____		_____ _____	
_____ _____		_____ _____	
_____ _____		_____ _____	
_____ _____		_____ _____	
_____ _____		_____ _____	
L _____ _____		S _____ _____	
_____ _____		_____ _____	
_____ _____		_____ _____	
_____ _____		_____ _____	
_____ _____		TOTAL CALORIES/POINTS _____	

Calories/Points Tracker

DAILY GOAL _____

FOODS	CALORIES/POINTS	FOODS	CALORIES/POINTS

FRI

B_____ _____

_____ _____

_____ _____

_____ _____

_____ _____

L_____ _____

_____ _____

_____ _____

_____ _____

_____ _____

D_____ _____

_____ _____

_____ _____

_____ _____

_____ _____

S_____ _____

_____ _____

_____ _____

_____ _____

TOTAL CALORIES/POINTS _____

FOODS	CALORIES/POINTS	FOODS	CALORIES/POINTS

SAT

B_____ _____

_____ _____

_____ _____

_____ _____

_____ _____

L_____ _____

_____ _____

_____ _____

_____ _____

_____ _____

D_____ _____

_____ _____

_____ _____

_____ _____

_____ _____

S_____ _____

_____ _____

_____ _____

_____ _____

TOTAL CALORIES/POINTS _____

DATE _____ / _____ / _____ TO _____ / _____ / _____

FOODS	CALORIES/ POINTS	FOODS	CALORIES/ POINTS
B _____	_____	D _____	_____
_____	_____	_____	_____
_____	_____	_____	_____
_____	_____	_____	_____
_____	_____	_____	_____
_____	_____	_____	_____
L _____	_____	S _____	_____
_____	_____	_____	_____
_____	_____	_____	_____
_____	_____	_____	_____
_____	_____		
_____	_____	TOTAL CALORIES/POINTS _____	

Exercise Tracker

ACTIVITY	DISTANCE/ DURATION/INTENSITY	CALORIES BURNED
_____	_____	_____
_____	_____	_____
_____	_____	_____
_____	_____	_____
_____	_____	_____
_____	_____	_____
_____	_____	_____
_____	_____	_____

Stuffed Chicken Breast with Pears and Brie

SERVES 4

- 2 large boneless, skinless chicken breasts (16 ounces total)
- ½ teaspoon plus a pinch of kosher salt

  Freshly ground black pepper
- 1 teaspoon olive oil
- ¼ cup chopped onion
- 2 slices prosciutto, chopped
- 1 pear, peeled and cut into ½-inch pieces
- 2 fresh sage leaves, chopped
- ¼ cup baby arugula
- 2 ounces Brie cheese, skin removed, divided

  Nonstick cooking spray

SERVING SIZE	½ stuffed breast
CALORIES	233
FAT	9 g
CHOLESTEROL	97 mg
CARBOHYDRATE	6 g
FIBER	1 g
PROTEIN	31 g
SUGAR	3.5 g
SODIUM	456 mg

Preheat the oven to 375°F.

Make a lengthwise cut into the side of the chicken breast to create a pocket for the stuffing. Season the inside and outside of the chicken with ½ teaspoon of the salt and pepper.

In a skillet set over medium heat, combine the oil, onions, and prosciutto. Cook, stirring, until golden, 3 to 4 minutes. Add the pear and sage, season with a pinch of salt, and cook until translucent, 3 to 4 minutes. Remove the pan from the heat and stir in the arugula. Set aside to cool for a few minutes.

Divide the pear mixture among the chicken breasts, stuffing each with the filling and the Brie. Using cooking twine, tie the breasts closed.

Heat an ovenproof skillet over medium-high heat and lightly coat with cooking spray. Sear the chicken on all sides except where the stuffing is, 3 to 4 minutes per side. Arrange the chicken in the skillet cut side up, cover tightly with foil, and place the skillet in the oven.

Bake until the chicken is cooked through, 23 to 25 minutes. Cut each breast in half and serve.

Weekly Meal Planner

Weekly Goals _____

_____

_____

_____

_____

superfood

BROCCOLI

Delicious cooked or raw, broccoli is
wonderful added to pastas, frittatas
and omelets, and salads, or eaten on
its own.

MON

TUE

WED

Calories/Points Tracker

DAILY GOAL

MON

FOODS	CALORIES/POINTS	FOODS	CALORIES/POINTS
B_____	____	D_____	____
_____	____	_____	____
_____	____	_____	____
_____	____	_____	____
_____	____	_____	____
_____	____	_____	____
L_____	____	S_____	____
_____	____	_____	____
_____	____	_____	____
_____	____	_____	____
_____	____	TOTAL CALORIES/POINTS ____
_____	____		

TUE

FOODS	CALORIES/POINTS	FOODS	CALORIES/POINTS
B_____	____	D_____	____
_____	____	_____	____
_____	____	_____	____
_____	____	_____	____
_____	____	_____	____
_____	____	_____	____
L_____	____	S_____	____
_____	____	_____	____
_____	____	_____	____
_____	____	_____	____
_____	____	TOTAL CALORIES/POINTS ____
_____	____		

DATE ____ / ____ / ____ TO ____ / ____ / ____

FOODS	CALORIES/ POINTS	FOODS	CALORIES/ POINTS
B _____	_____	D _____	_____
_____	_____	_____	_____
_____	_____	_____	_____
_____	_____	_____	_____
_____	_____	_____	_____
_____	_____	_____	_____
L _____	_____	S _____	_____
_____	_____	_____	_____
_____	_____	_____	_____
_____	_____	_____	_____
_____	_____	_____	_____
_____	_____	TOTAL CALORIES/POINTS _____	

FOODS	CALORIES/ POINTS	FOODS	CALORIES/ POINTS
B _____	_____	D _____	_____
_____	_____	_____	_____
_____	_____	_____	_____
_____	_____	_____	_____
_____	_____	_____	_____
_____	_____	_____	_____
L _____	_____	S _____	_____
_____	_____	_____	_____
_____	_____	_____	_____
_____	_____	_____	_____
_____	_____	_____	_____
_____	_____	TOTAL CALORIES/POINTS _____	

Calories/Points Tracker

DAILY GOAL

FRI

FOODS	CALORIES/POINTS	FOODS	CALORIES/POINTS
B_____	_____	D_____	_____
_____	_____	_____	_____
_____	_____	_____	_____
_____	_____	_____	_____
_____	_____	_____	_____
_____	_____	_____	_____
L_____	_____	S_____	_____
_____	_____	_____	_____
_____	_____	_____	_____
_____	_____	_____	_____
_____	_____		
_____	_____	TOTAL CALORIES/POINTS _____	

SAT

FOODS	CALORIES/POINTS	FOODS	CALORIES/POINTS
B_____	_____	D_____	_____
_____	_____	_____	_____
_____	_____	_____	_____
_____	_____	_____	_____
_____	_____	_____	_____
_____	_____	_____	_____
L_____	_____	S_____	_____
_____	_____	_____	_____
_____	_____	_____	_____
_____	_____	_____	_____
_____	_____		
_____	_____	TOTAL CALORIES/POINTS _____	

DATE _____ / _____ / _____ TO _____ / _____ / _____

FOODS	CALORIES/ POINTS	FOODS	CALORIES/ POINTS
B_____	_____	D_____	_____
_____	_____	_____	_____
_____	_____	_____	_____
_____	_____	_____	_____
_____	_____	_____	_____
_____	_____	_____	_____
L_____	_____	S_____	_____
_____	_____	_____	_____
_____	_____	_____	_____
_____	_____	_____	_____
_____	_____	TOTAL CALORIES/POINTS _____	
_____	_____		

--------- Exercise Tracker ---------

ACTIVITY	DISTANCE/ DURATION/INTENSITY	CALORIES BURNED
_____	_____	_____
_____	_____	_____
_____	_____	_____
_____	_____	_____
_____	_____	_____
_____	_____	_____
_____	_____	_____
_____	_____	_____

Weekly Meal Planner

Weekly Goals _____

_____

_____

_____

_____

> "Life shrinks
> or expands in
> proportion to one's
> courage."
>
> **ANAïS NIN**

MON

_____
_____
_____
_____
_____

TUE

_____
_____
_____
_____
_____

WED

_____
_____
_____
_____
_____

Calories/Points Tracker

MON

FOODS	CALORIES/POINTS
B_____	_____
_____	_____
_____	_____
_____	_____
_____	_____
_____	_____
L_____	_____
_____	_____
_____	_____
_____	_____
_____	_____
_____	_____

FOODS	CALORIES/POINTS
D_____	_____
_____	_____
_____	_____
_____	_____
_____	_____
_____	_____
S_____	_____
_____	_____
_____	_____
_____	_____
TOTAL CALORIES/POINTS	_____

TUE

FOODS	CALORIES/POINTS
B_____	_____
_____	_____
_____	_____
_____	_____
_____	_____
_____	_____
L_____	_____
_____	_____
_____	_____
_____	_____
_____	_____
_____	_____

FOODS	CALORIES/POINTS
D_____	_____
_____	_____
_____	_____
_____	_____
_____	_____
_____	_____
S_____	_____
_____	_____
_____	_____
_____	_____
TOTAL CALORIES/POINTS	_____

DATE ___ / ___ / ___ TO ___ / ___ / ___

FOODS	CALORIES/POINTS	FOODS	CALORIES/POINTS
B_____	____	D_____	____
_____	____	_____	____
_____	____	_____	____
_____	____	_____	____
_____	____	_____	____
_____	____	_____	____
L_____	____	S_____	____
_____	____	_____	____
_____	____	_____	____
_____	____	_____	____
_____	____	TOTAL CALORIES/POINTS ____
_____	____		

FOODS	CALORIES/POINTS	FOODS	CALORIES/POINTS
B_____	____	D_____	____
_____	____	_____	____
_____	____	_____	____
_____	____	_____	____
_____	____	_____	____
_____	____	_____	____
L_____	____	S_____	____
_____	____	_____	____
_____	____	_____	____
_____	____	_____	____
_____	____	TOTAL CALORIES/POINTS ____

Calories/Points Tracker

DAILY GOAL

FRI

FOODS	CALORIES/ POINTS	FOODS	CALORIES/ POINTS
B_____	_____	D_____	_____
_____	_____	_____	_____
_____	_____	_____	_____
_____	_____	_____	_____
_____	_____	_____	_____
_____	_____	_____	_____
L_____	_____	S_____	_____
_____	_____	_____	_____
_____	_____	_____	_____
_____	_____	_____	_____
_____	_____		
_____	_____	TOTAL CALORIES/POINTS _____	

SAT

FOODS	CALORIES/ POINTS	FOODS	CALORIES/ POINTS
B_____	_____	D_____	_____
_____	_____	_____	_____
_____	_____	_____	_____
_____	_____	_____	_____
_____	_____	_____	_____
_____	_____	_____	_____
L_____	_____	S_____	_____
_____	_____	_____	_____
_____	_____	_____	_____
_____	_____	_____	_____
_____	_____		
_____	_____	TOTAL CALORIES/POINTS _____	

DATE ___ / ___ / ___ TO ___ / ___ / ___

FOODS	CALORIES/ POINTS	FOODS	CALORIES/ POINTS
B _____	___	D _____	___
_____	___	_____	___
_____	___	_____	___
_____	___	_____	___
_____	___	_____	___
_____	___	_____	___
L _____	___	S _____	___
_____	___	_____	___
_____	___	_____	___
_____	___	_____	___
_____	___	TOTAL CALORIES/POINTS ___	
_____	___		

―――――――――― Exercise Tracker ――――――――――

ACTIVITY	DISTANCE/ DURATION/INTENSITY	CALORIES BURNED
_____	_____	_____
_____	_____	_____
_____	_____	_____
_____	_____	_____
_____	_____	_____
_____	_____	_____
_____	_____	_____
_____	_____	_____

Weekly Meal Planner

Weekly Goals _____

_____

_____

_____

_____

MON

TUE

WED

THU

FRI

SAT

SUN

Calories/Points Tracker

MON

FOODS	CALORIES/POINTS
B_____	_____
_____	_____
_____	_____
_____	_____
_____	_____
_____	_____
L_____	_____
_____	_____
_____	_____
_____	_____
_____	_____
_____	_____

FOODS	CALORIES/POINTS
D_____	_____
_____	_____
_____	_____
_____	_____
_____	_____
S_____	_____
_____	_____
_____	_____
_____	_____
TOTAL CALORIES/POINTS	_____

TUE

FOODS	CALORIES/POINTS
B_____	_____
_____	_____
_____	_____
_____	_____
_____	_____
_____	_____
L_____	_____
_____	_____
_____	_____
_____	_____
_____	_____
_____	_____

FOODS	CALORIES/POINTS
D_____	_____
_____	_____
_____	_____
_____	_____
_____	_____
S_____	_____
_____	_____
_____	_____
_____	_____
TOTAL CALORIES/POINTS	_____

DATE ___ / ___ / ___ TO ___ / ___ / ___

FOODS	CALORIES/ POINTS	FOODS	CALORIES/ POINTS
B		D	
L		S	
		TOTAL CALORIES/POINTS _____	

FOODS	CALORIES/ POINTS	FOODS	CALORIES/ POINTS
B		D	
L		S	
		TOTAL CALORIES/POINTS _____	

Calories/Points Tracker

DAILY GOAL _____

FRI

FOODS	CALORIES/POINTS
B _____	_____
_____	_____
_____	_____
_____	_____
_____	_____
_____	_____
L _____	_____
_____	_____
_____	_____
_____	_____
_____	_____
_____	_____

FOODS	CALORIES/POINTS
D _____	_____
_____	_____
_____	_____
_____	_____
_____	_____
_____	_____
S _____	_____
_____	_____
_____	_____
_____	_____

TOTAL CALORIES/POINTS _____

SAT

FOODS	CALORIES/POINTS
B _____	_____
_____	_____
_____	_____
_____	_____
_____	_____
_____	_____
L _____	_____
_____	_____
_____	_____
_____	_____
_____	_____
_____	_____

FOODS	CALORIES/POINTS
D _____	_____
_____	_____
_____	_____
_____	_____
_____	_____
_____	_____
S _____	_____
_____	_____
_____	_____
_____	_____

TOTAL CALORIES/POINTS _____

DATE ___/___/___ TO ___/___/___

FOODS	CALORIES/POINTS	FOODS	CALORIES/POINTS
B_____	____	D_____	____
_____	____	_____	____
_____	____	_____	____
_____	____	_____	____
_____	____	_____	____
_____	____	_____	____
L_____	____	S_____	____
_____	____	_____	____
_____	____	_____	____
_____	____	_____	____
_____	____	TOTAL CALORIES/POINTS ____
_____	____		

Exercise Tracker

ACTIVITY	DISTANCE/DURATION/INTENSITY	CALORIES BURNED
_____	_____	_____
_____	_____	_____
_____	_____	_____
_____	_____	_____
_____	_____	_____
_____	_____	_____
_____	_____	_____
_____	_____	_____

Broccoli-and-Cheese Tots

MAKES ABOUT 28 TOTS; SERVES 4

Nonstick cooking spray

12 ounces broccoli florets

1 large egg

1 large egg white

2/3 cup grated reduced-fat sharp
 cheddar cheese

1/2 cup finely chopped scallions

1/2 cup seasoned breadcrumbs

1/4 teaspoon kosher salt

Freshly ground black pepper

SERVING SIZE	7 tots
CALORIES	152
FAT	6 g
CHOLESTEROL	47 mg
CARBOHYDRATE	14 g
FIBER	4 g
PROTEIN	12.5 g
SUGAR	1 g
SODIUM	485.5 mg

Preheat the oven to 400°F. Spray a nonstick baking sheet with nonstick cooking spray.

Blanch the broccoli in a pot of boiling water for 1 minute, drain, rinse under cold water, and drain again. Pat dry with paper towels. Finely chop the broccoli and put 2 cups in a medium bowl. Add the egg, egg white, cheese, scallions, breadcrumbs, and salt, and season with pepper to taste. Spoon heaping tablespoons of the mixture into your hand and roll into small ovals. Place them on the prepared baking sheet.

Bake in the oven until golden, turning halfway, 16 to 18 minutes.

Slow Cooker Applesauce

MAKES 3 CUPS; SERVES 12

8 medium apples, a combination of Golden Delicious, Honey Crisp, Fuji, and/or Gala

1 (3-inch) cinnamon stick

1 strip lemon zest

1 teaspoon fresh lemon juice

5 teaspoons light brown sugar, unpacked

SERVING SIZE	¼ cup
CALORIES	55
FAT	0 g
CHOLESTEROL	0 mg
CARBOHYDRATE	15 g
FIBER	2 g
PROTEIN	0 g
SUGAR	12 g
SODIUM	0.5 mg

Peel, core, and slice the apples. Place them in the slow cooker. Add the cinnamon stick, lemon zest, lemon juice, and brown sugar.

Set the slow cooker to Low, cover, and cook until the apples are soft throughout, 6 hours. Stir apples occasionally. Remove the cinnamon stick and use an immersion blender to blend until smooth, or if you prefer a chunky sauce, skip the blender.

Weekly Meal Planner

Weekly Goals _____

_____

_____

_____

_____

superfood

SALMON

Salmon is really easy to prepare—
trust me! And leftovers are
delicious the next day served
chilled and with a salad.

MON

TUE

WED

Calories/Points Tracker

DAILY GOAL

MON

FOODS CALORIES/POINTS

B _____ _____
_____ _____
_____ _____
_____ _____
_____ _____
_____ _____

L _____ _____
_____ _____
_____ _____
_____ _____
_____ _____
_____ _____

FOODS CALORIES/POINTS

D _____ _____
_____ _____
_____ _____
_____ _____
_____ _____

S _____ _____
_____ _____
_____ _____
_____ _____

TOTAL CALORIES/POINTS _____

TUE

FOODS CALORIES/POINTS

B _____ _____
_____ _____
_____ _____
_____ _____
_____ _____
_____ _____

L _____ _____
_____ _____
_____ _____
_____ _____
_____ _____
_____ _____

FOODS CALORIES/POINTS

D _____ _____
_____ _____
_____ _____
_____ _____
_____ _____

S _____ _____
_____ _____
_____ _____
_____ _____

TOTAL CALORIES/POINTS _____

DATE ___ / ___ / ___ TO ___ / ___ / ___

FOODS	CALORIES/ POINTS	FOODS	CALORIES/ POINTS
B_____	_____	D_____	_____
_____	_____	_____	_____
_____	_____	_____	_____
_____	_____	_____	_____
_____	_____	_____	_____
_____	_____	_____	_____
L_____	_____	S_____	_____
_____	_____	_____	_____
_____	_____	_____	_____
_____	_____	_____	_____
_____	_____		
_____	_____	TOTAL CALORIES/POINTS _____	

FOODS	CALORIES/ POINTS	FOODS	CALORIES/ POINTS
B_____	_____	D_____	_____
_____	_____	_____	_____
_____	_____	_____	_____
_____	_____	_____	_____
_____	_____	_____	_____
_____	_____	_____	_____
L_____	_____	S_____	_____
_____	_____	_____	_____
_____	_____	_____	_____
_____	_____	_____	_____
_____	_____		
_____	_____	TOTAL CALORIES/POINTS _____	

Calories/Points Tracker

DAILY GOAL _____

FRI

FOODS	CALORIES/POINTS
B_____	_____
_____	_____
_____	_____
_____	_____
_____	_____
_____	_____
L_____	_____
_____	_____
_____	_____
_____	_____
_____	_____

FOODS	CALORIES/POINTS
D_____	_____
_____	_____
_____	_____
_____	_____
_____	_____
S_____	_____
_____	_____
_____	_____
_____	_____

TOTAL CALORIES/POINTS _____

SAT

FOODS	CALORIES/POINTS
B_____	_____
_____	_____
_____	_____
_____	_____
_____	_____
L_____	_____
_____	_____
_____	_____
_____	_____
_____	_____

FOODS	CALORIES/POINTS
D_____	_____
_____	_____
_____	_____
_____	_____
_____	_____
S_____	_____
_____	_____
_____	_____
_____	_____

TOTAL CALORIES/POINTS _____

DATE ___ / ___ / ___ TO ___ / ___ / ___

FOODS	CALORIES/ POINTS	FOODS	CALORIES/ POINTS
B_____ ____		D_____ ____	
_____ ____		_____ ____	
_____ ____		_____ ____	
_____ ____		_____ ____	
_____ ____		_____ ____	
_____ ____		_____ ____	
L_____ ____		S_____ ____	
_____ ____		_____ ____	
_____ ____		_____ ____	
_____ ____		_____ ____	
_____ ____			
_____ ____		TOTAL CALORIES/POINTS ____	

—————————— Exercise Tracker ——————————

ACTIVITY	DISTANCE/ DURATION/INTENSITY	CALORIES BURNED
_____	_____	_____
_____	_____	_____
_____	_____	_____
_____	_____	_____
_____	_____	_____
_____	_____	_____
_____	_____	_____
_____	_____	_____

Weekly Meal Planner

Weekly Goals _____

_____

_____

_____

_____

MON

_____

_____

_____

_____

TUE

_____

_____

_____

_____

WED

_____

_____

_____

Calories/Points Tracker

DAILY GOAL _____

MON

FOODS	CALORIES/ POINTS	FOODS	CALORIES/ POINTS
B_____	_____	D_____	_____
_____	_____	_____	_____
_____	_____	_____	_____
_____	_____	_____	_____
_____	_____	_____	_____
_____	_____	_____	_____
L_____	_____	S_____	_____
_____	_____	_____	_____
_____	_____	_____	_____
_____	_____	_____	_____
_____	_____	_____	_____
_____	_____	TOTAL CALORIES/POINTS _____	

TUE

FOODS	CALORIES/ POINTS	FOODS	CALORIES/ POINTS
B_____	_____	D_____	_____
_____	_____	_____	_____
_____	_____	_____	_____
_____	_____	_____	_____
_____	_____	_____	_____
_____	_____	_____	_____
L_____	_____	S_____	_____
_____	_____	_____	_____
_____	_____	_____	_____
_____	_____	_____	_____
_____	_____	_____	_____
_____	_____	TOTAL CALORIES/POINTS _____	

DATE ____ / ____ / ____ TO ____ / ____ / ____

FOODS	CALORIES/ POINTS	FOODS	CALORIES/ POINTS
B _____ _____		D _____ _____	
_____ _____		_____ _____	
_____ _____		_____ _____	
_____ _____		_____ _____	
_____ _____		_____ _____	
_____ _____		_____ _____	
L _____ _____		S _____ _____	
_____ _____		_____ _____	
_____ _____		_____ _____	
_____ _____		_____ _____	
_____ _____			
_____ _____		TOTAL CALORIES/POINTS _____	

FOODS	CALORIES/ POINTS	FOODS	CALORIES/ POINTS
B _____ _____		D _____ _____	
_____ _____		_____ _____	
_____ _____		_____ _____	
_____ _____		_____ _____	
_____ _____		_____ _____	
_____ _____		_____ _____	
L _____ _____		S _____ _____	
_____ _____		_____ _____	
_____ _____		_____ _____	
_____ _____		_____ _____	
_____ _____			
_____ _____		TOTAL CALORIES/POINTS _____	

Calories/Points Tracker

DAILY GOAL

FOODS	CALORIES/POINTS	FOODS	CALORIES/POINTS
B_____	_____	D_____	_____
_____	_____	_____	_____
_____	_____	_____	_____
_____	_____	_____	_____
_____	_____	_____	_____
_____	_____	_____	_____
L_____	_____	S_____	_____
_____	_____	_____	_____
_____	_____	_____	_____
_____	_____	_____	_____
_____	_____		
_____	_____	TOTAL CALORIES/POINTS _____	

FRI

FOODS	CALORIES/POINTS	FOODS	CALORIES/POINTS
B_____	_____	D_____	_____
_____	_____	_____	_____
_____	_____	_____	_____
_____	_____	_____	_____
_____	_____	_____	_____
_____	_____	_____	_____
L_____	_____	S_____	_____
_____	_____	_____	_____
_____	_____	_____	_____
_____	_____	_____	_____
_____	_____		
_____	_____	TOTAL CALORIES/POINTS _____	

SAT

DATE ____ / ____ / ____ TO ____ / ____ / ____

FOODS	CALORIES/POINTS	FOODS	CALORIES/POINTS
B _____	_____	D _____	_____
_____	_____	_____	_____
_____	_____	_____	_____
_____	_____	_____	_____
_____	_____	_____	_____
_____	_____	_____	_____
L _____	_____	S _____	_____
_____	_____	_____	_____
_____	_____	_____	_____
_____	_____	_____	_____
_____	_____	TOTAL CALORIES/POINTS _____
_____	_____		

—————————————————— Exercise Tracker ——————————————————

ACTIVITY	DISTANCE/DURATION/INTENSITY	CALORIES BURNED
_____	_____	_____
_____	_____	_____
_____	_____	_____
_____	_____	_____
_____	_____	_____
_____	_____	_____
_____	_____	_____

Weekly Meal Planner

Weekly Goals _____

_____

_____

_____

_____

superfood

YOGURT

Yogurt is one of the quickest breakfasts you can eat, and you can mix in other healthy foods like berries and fruit, granola, or a little honey.

MON

TUE

WED

Calories/Points Tracker

MON

FOODS	CALORIES/POINTS
B _____	_____
_____	_____
_____	_____
_____	_____
_____	_____
_____	_____
L _____	_____
_____	_____
_____	_____
_____	_____
_____	_____

FOODS	CALORIES/POINTS
D _____	_____
_____	_____
_____	_____
_____	_____
_____	_____
_____	_____
S _____	_____
_____	_____
_____	_____
_____	_____
TOTAL CALORIES/POINTS	_____

TUE

FOODS	CALORIES/POINTS
B _____	_____
_____	_____
_____	_____
_____	_____
_____	_____
_____	_____
L _____	_____
_____	_____
_____	_____
_____	_____
_____	_____

FOODS	CALORIES/POINTS
D _____	_____
_____	_____
_____	_____
_____	_____
_____	_____
_____	_____
S _____	_____
_____	_____
_____	_____
_____	_____
TOTAL CALORIES/POINTS	_____

WED

FOODS	CALORIES/ POINTS	FOODS	CALORIES/ POINTS
B_____	_____	D_____	_____
_____	_____	_____	_____
_____	_____	_____	_____
_____	_____	_____	_____
_____	_____	_____	_____
_____	_____	_____	_____
L_____	_____	S_____	_____
_____	_____	_____	_____
_____	_____	_____	_____
_____	_____	_____	_____
_____	_____		
_____	_____	TOTAL CALORIES/POINTS _____	

THU

FOODS	CALORIES/ POINTS	FOODS	CALORIES/ POINTS
B_____	_____	D_____	_____
_____	_____	_____	_____
_____	_____	_____	_____
_____	_____	_____	_____
_____	_____	_____	_____
_____	_____	_____	_____
L_____	_____	S_____	_____
_____	_____	_____	_____
_____	_____	_____	_____
_____	_____	_____	_____
_____	_____		
_____	_____	TOTAL CALORIES/POINTS _____	

Calories/Points Tracker

FRI

FOODS	CALORIES/ POINTS	FOODS	CALORIES/ POINTS
B_____	_____	D_____	_____
_____	_____	_____	_____
_____	_____	_____	_____
_____	_____	_____	_____
_____	_____	_____	_____
_____	_____	_____	_____
L_____	_____	S_____	_____
_____	_____	_____	_____
_____	_____	_____	_____
_____	_____	_____	_____
_____	_____		
_____	_____	TOTAL CALORIES/POINTS _____	

SAT

FOODS	CALORIES/ POINTS	FOODS	CALORIES/ POINTS
B_____	_____	D_____	_____
_____	_____	_____	_____
_____	_____	_____	_____
_____	_____	_____	_____
_____	_____	_____	_____
_____	_____	_____	_____
L_____	_____	S_____	_____
_____	_____	_____	_____
_____	_____	_____	_____
_____	_____	_____	_____
_____	_____		
_____	_____	TOTAL CALORIES/POINTS _____	

SUN

DATE ___/___/___ TO ___/___/___

FOODS	CALORIES/POINTS	FOODS	CALORIES/POINTS
B_____	____	D_____	____
_____	____	_____	____
_____	____	_____	____
_____	____	_____	____
_____	____	_____	____
_____	____	_____	____
L_____	____	S_____	____
_____	____	_____	____
_____	____	_____	____
_____	____	_____	____
_____	____		
_____	____	TOTAL CALORIES/POINTS _____	

———————— Exercise Tracker ————————

ACTIVITY	DISTANCE/DURATION/INTENSITY	CALORIES BURNED
_____	_____	_____
_____	_____	_____
_____	_____	_____
_____	_____	_____
_____	_____	_____
_____	_____	_____
_____	_____	_____

Grilled Garlic-Dijon-Herb Salmon

SERVES 4

- 4 garlic cloves
- 2 tablespoons Dijon mustard
- 1 teaspoon olive oil
- 1 teaspoon red wine vinegar
- 1 teaspoon Herbs de Provence dried herb mix
- 4 (6-ounce) wild salmon fillets, 1-inch thick (if frozen, thaw first)
- ¼ teaspoon kosher salt
- Freshly ground black pepper
- Olive oil spray (I use my Misto)
- 4 lemon wedges, for serving

SERVING SIZE	1 fillet with lemon
CALORIES	233.5
FAT	8 g
CHOLESTEROL	127.5 mg
CARBOHYDRATE	3 g
FIBER	0 g
PROTEIN	35 g
SUGAR	0 g
SODIUM	310.5 mg

In a mini food processor, or using a mortar and pestle, mash the garlic, mustard, oil, vinegar, and Herbs de Provence until the mixture becomes a paste. Set aside.

Season the salmon with the salt and pepper. Heat a grill or grill pan over high heat until hot. Spray the pan lightly with oil and reduce the heat to medium-low. Place the salmon on the hot pan and cook, without moving, until golden, 4 minutes. Flip the salmon and cook until the second side is golden, 4 minutes. Spoon half of the mustard sauce on top of the fillets. Flip the salmon again and cook 1 more minute, spooning the remaining sauce over the fillets. Turn once again and cook until cooked through, about 1 more minute. (The fish should have a total cooking time of 9 to 10 minutes per inch thickness.)

Transfer the fillets to plates and serve with fresh lemon wedges.

Weekly Meal Planner

Weekly Goals _____

_____

_____

_____

_____

"Challenges are what
make life interesting;
overcoming them
is what makes life
meaningful."

JOSHUA J. MARINE

MON

TUE

WED

Calories/Points Tracker

MON

FOODS	CALORIES/ POINTS
B _____	____
_____	____
_____	____
_____	____
_____	____
_____	____
L _____	____
_____	____
_____	____
_____	____
_____	____
_____	____

FOODS	CALORIES/ POINTS
D _____	____
_____	____
_____	____
_____	____
_____	____
_____	____
S _____	____
_____	____
_____	____
_____	____
TOTAL CALORIES/POINTS	____

TUE

FOODS	CALORIES/ POINTS
B _____	____
_____	____
_____	____
_____	____
_____	____
_____	____
L _____	____
_____	____
_____	____
_____	____
_____	____
_____	____

FOODS	CALORIES/ POINTS
D _____	____
_____	____
_____	____
_____	____
_____	____
_____	____
S _____	____
_____	____
_____	____
_____	____
TOTAL CALORIES/POINTS	____

DATE ___ / ___ / ___ TO ___ / ___ / ___

FOODS	CALORIES/ POINTS	FOODS	CALORIES/ POINTS
B_____	___	D_____	___
_____	___	_____	___
_____	___	_____	___
_____	___	_____	___
_____	___	_____	___
_____	___	_____	___
L_____	___	S_____	___
_____	___	_____	___
_____	___	_____	___
_____	___	_____	___
_____	___	_____	___
_____	___	TOTAL CALORIES/POINTS ___	

FOODS	CALORIES/ POINTS	FOODS	CALORIES/ POINTS
B_____	___	D_____	___
_____	___	_____	___
_____	___	_____	___
_____	___	_____	___
_____	___	_____	___
_____	___	_____	___
L_____	___	S_____	___
_____	___	_____	___
_____	___	_____	___
_____	___	_____	___
_____	___	TOTAL CALORIES/POINTS ___	

Calories/Points Tracker

FRI

FOODS	CALORIES/POINTS	FOODS	CALORIES/POINTS
B_____ _____		D_____ _____	
_____ _____		_____ _____	
_____ _____		_____ _____	
_____ _____		_____ _____	
_____ _____		_____ _____	
_____ _____		_____ _____	
L_____ _____		S_____ _____	
_____ _____		_____ _____	
_____ _____		_____ _____	
_____ _____		_____ _____	
_____ _____			
_____ _____			

TOTAL CALORIES/POINTS _____

SAT

FOODS	CALORIES/POINTS	FOODS	CALORIES/POINTS
B_____ _____		D_____ _____	
_____ _____		_____ _____	
_____ _____		_____ _____	
_____ _____		_____ _____	
_____ _____		_____ _____	
_____ _____		_____ _____	
L_____ _____		S_____ _____	
_____ _____		_____ _____	
_____ _____		_____ _____	
_____ _____		_____ _____	
_____ _____			
_____ _____			

TOTAL CALORIES/POINTS _____

DATE ___ / ___ / ___ TO ___ / ___ / ___

FOODS	CALORIES/ POINTS	FOODS	CALORIES/ POINTS
B _____	___	D _____	___
_____	___	_____	___
_____	___	_____	___
_____	___	_____	___
_____	___	_____	___
_____	___	_____	___
L _____	___	S _____	___
_____	___	_____	___
_____	___	_____	___
_____	___	_____	___
_____	___		
_____	___	TOTAL CALORIES/POINTS ___	

——————————— Exercise Tracker ———————————

ACTIVITY	DISTANCE/ DURATION/INTENSITY	CALORIES BURNED
_____	_____	_____
_____	_____	_____
_____	_____	_____
_____	_____	_____
_____	_____	_____
_____	_____	_____
_____	_____	_____
_____	_____	_____

Weekly Meal Planner

Weekly Goals _____

_____

_____

_____

_____

> "If you want to lift yourself up, lift up someone else."
>
> BOOKER T. WASHINGTON

MON

TUE

WED

Calories/Points Tracker

MON

FOODS	CALORIES/ POINTS
B_____	_____
_____	_____
_____	_____
_____	_____
_____	_____
_____	_____
L_____	_____
_____	_____
_____	_____
_____	_____
_____	_____
_____	_____

FOODS	CALORIES/ POINTS
D_____	_____
_____	_____
_____	_____
_____	_____
_____	_____
S_____	_____
_____	_____
_____	_____
_____	_____
TOTAL CALORIES/POINTS	_____

TUE

FOODS	CALORIES/ POINTS
B_____	_____
_____	_____
_____	_____
_____	_____
_____	_____
_____	_____
L_____	_____
_____	_____
_____	_____
_____	_____
_____	_____
_____	_____

FOODS	CALORIES/ POINTS
D_____	_____
_____	_____
_____	_____
_____	_____
_____	_____
S_____	_____
_____	_____
_____	_____
_____	_____
TOTAL CALORIES/POINTS	_____

DATE _____ / _____ / _____ TO _____ / _____ / _____

FOODS	CALORIES/POINTS	FOODS	CALORIES/POINTS
B_____ ____		D_____ ____	
_____ ____		_____ ____	
_____ ____		_____ ____	
_____ ____		_____ ____	
_____ ____		_____ ____	
_____ ____		_____ ____	
L_____ ____		S_____ ____	
_____ ____		_____ ____	
_____ ____		_____ ____	
_____ ____		_____ ____	
_____ ____		TOTAL CALORIES/POINTS ____	

FOODS	CALORIES/POINTS	FOODS	CALORIES/POINTS
B_____ ____		D_____ ____	
_____ ____		_____ ____	
_____ ____		_____ ____	
_____ ____		_____ ____	
_____ ____		_____ ____	
_____ ____		_____ ____	
L_____ ____		S_____ ____	
_____ ____		_____ ____	
_____ ____		_____ ____	
_____ ____		_____ ____	
_____ ____		TOTAL CALORIES/POINTS ____	

Calories/Points Tracker

DAILY GOAL

FRI

FOODS	CALORIES/POINTS	FOODS	CALORIES/POINTS
B _____	_____	D _____	_____
_____	_____	_____	_____
_____	_____	_____	_____
_____	_____	_____	_____
_____	_____	_____	_____
_____	_____	_____	_____
L _____	_____	S _____	_____
_____	_____	_____	_____
_____	_____	_____	_____
_____	_____	_____	_____
_____	_____		
_____	_____	TOTAL CALORIES/POINTS _____

SAT

FOODS	CALORIES/POINTS	FOODS	CALORIES/POINTS
B _____	_____	D _____	_____
_____	_____	_____	_____
_____	_____	_____	_____
_____	_____	_____	_____
_____	_____	_____	_____
_____	_____	_____	_____
L _____	_____	S _____	_____
_____	_____	_____	_____
_____	_____	_____	_____
_____	_____	_____	_____
_____	_____		
_____	_____	TOTAL CALORIES/POINTS _____

DATE _____ / _____ / _____ TO _____ / _____ / _____

FOODS	CALORIES/ POINTS	FOODS	CALORIES/ POINTS
B_____	_____	D_____	_____
_____	_____	_____	_____
_____	_____	_____	_____
_____	_____	_____	_____
_____	_____	_____	_____
_____	_____	_____	_____
L_____	_____	S_____	_____
_____	_____	_____	_____
_____	_____	_____	_____
_____	_____	_____	_____
_____	_____		
_____	_____	TOTAL CALORIES/POINTS _____

—————————————— Exercise Tracker ——————————————

ACTIVITY	DISTANCE/ DURATION/INTENSITY	CALORIES BURNED
_____	_____	_____
_____	_____	_____
_____	_____	_____
_____	_____	_____
_____	_____	_____
_____	_____	_____
_____	_____	_____
_____	_____	_____

Weekly Meal Planner

Weekly Goals _____

_____

_____

_____

_____

superfood

KALE

You can do more with kale than make a salad! Try sautéing it with garlic for a side dish or adding it to frittatas and omelets.

MON

TUE

WED

Calories/Points Tracker

DAILY GOAL _____

MON

FOODS · CALORIES/POINTS

B _____ _____
_____ _____
_____ _____
_____ _____
_____ _____
_____ _____

L _____ _____
_____ _____
_____ _____
_____ _____
_____ _____
_____ _____

FOODS · CALORIES/POINTS

D _____ _____
_____ _____
_____ _____
_____ _____
_____ _____
_____ _____

S _____ _____
_____ _____
_____ _____
_____ _____

TOTAL CALORIES/POINTS _____

TUE

FOODS · CALORIES/POINTS

B _____ _____
_____ _____
_____ _____
_____ _____
_____ _____
_____ _____

L _____ _____
_____ _____
_____ _____
_____ _____
_____ _____
_____ _____

FOODS · CALORIES/POINTS

D _____ _____
_____ _____
_____ _____
_____ _____
_____ _____
_____ _____

S _____ _____
_____ _____
_____ _____
_____ _____

TOTAL CALORIES/POINTS _____

DATE ____ / ____ / ____ TO ____ / ____ / ____

FOODS	CALORIES/ POINTS	FOODS	CALORIES/ POINTS
B_____	_____	D_____	_____
_____	_____	_____	_____
_____	_____	_____	_____
_____	_____	_____	_____
_____	_____	_____	_____
_____	_____	_____	_____
L_____	_____	S_____	_____
_____	_____	_____	_____
_____	_____	_____	_____
_____	_____	_____	_____
_____	_____		
_____	_____	TOTAL CALORIES/POINTS _____	

FOODS	CALORIES/ POINTS	FOODS	CALORIES/ POINTS
B_____	_____	D_____	_____
_____	_____	_____	_____
_____	_____	_____	_____
_____	_____	_____	_____
_____	_____	_____	_____
_____	_____	_____	_____
L_____	_____	S_____	_____
_____	_____	_____	_____
_____	_____	_____	_____
_____	_____	_____	_____
_____	_____		
_____	_____	TOTAL CALORIES/POINTS _____	

Calories/Points Tracker

DAILY GOAL _____

FRI

FOODS	CALORIES/POINTS	FOODS	CALORIES/POINTS
B_____ _____		D_____ _____	
_____ _____		_____ _____	
_____ _____		_____ _____	
_____ _____		_____ _____	
_____ _____		_____ _____	
L_____ _____		S_____ _____	
_____ _____		_____ _____	
_____ _____		_____ _____	
_____ _____		_____ _____	
_____ _____		TOTAL CALORIES/POINTS _____	

SAT

FOODS	CALORIES/POINTS	FOODS	CALORIES/POINTS
B_____ _____		D_____ _____	
_____ _____		_____ _____	
_____ _____		_____ _____	
_____ _____		_____ _____	
_____ _____		_____ _____	
L_____ _____		S_____ _____	
_____ _____		_____ _____	
_____ _____		_____ _____	
_____ _____		_____ _____	
_____ _____		TOTAL CALORIES/POINTS _____	

DATE ___ / ___ / ___ TO ___ / ___ / ___

FOODS	CALORIES/ POINTS	FOODS	CALORIES/ POINTS
B _____	___	D _____	___
_____	___	_____	___
_____	___	_____	___
_____	___	_____	___
_____	___	_____	___
_____	___	_____	___
L _____	___	S _____	___
_____	___	_____	___
_____	___	_____	___
_____	___	_____	___
_____	___	TOTAL CALORIES/POINTS ___
_____	___		

— Exercise Tracker —

ACTIVITY	DISTANCE/ DURATION/INTENSITY	CALORIES BURNED
_____	_____	_____
_____	_____	_____
_____	_____	_____
_____	_____	_____
_____	_____	_____
_____	_____	_____
_____	_____	_____
_____	_____	_____

Grilled Stone Fruit Salad with Honey–Goat Cheese Dressing

MAKES 4 SALADS; SERVES 4

FOR THE DRESSING

- 2.5 ounces fresh creamy goat cheese, room temperature
- 1 tablespoon honey
- ½ tablespoon extra-virgin olive oil
- 2 teaspoons fresh lemon juice
- 1½ teaspoons apple cider vinegar
- 1½ tablespoons water
- ⅛ teaspoon kosher salt

  Freshly ground black pepper

SERVING SIZE	1 salad
CALORIES	202
FAT	14 g
CHOLESTEROL	8 mg
CARBOHYDRATE	16.5 g
FIBER	3 g
PROTEIN	6.5 g
SUGAR	13 g
SODIUM	122.5 mg

FOR THE SALAD

  Olive oil spray (I use my Misto)
- 2 ripe medium peaches, halved and sliced into wedges
- 2 medium ripe plums, halved and sliced into wedges
- 6 cups mixed baby greens
- 24 walnut or pecan halves

In a blender, combine the goat cheese, honey, olive oil, lemon juice, vinegar, and water and season with the salt and pepper. Blend well and refrigerate until ready to use.

Heat a grill pan over medium-high heat. Spray lightly with oil and grill the fruit until char marks form, about 1 minute.

Divide the greens among four plates, top with the grilled fruit and nuts, and drizzle 2 tablespoons of dressing over each.

Weekly Meal Planner

Weekly Goals _____

_____

_____

_____

_____

"Limitations live
only in our minds."

JAMIE PAOLINETTI

MON

TUE

WED

THU

FRI

SAT

SUN

Calories/Points Tracker

DAILY GOAL _____

MON

FOODS	CALORIES/POINTS	FOODS	CALORIES/POINTS
B_____	_____	D_____	_____
_____	_____	_____	_____
_____	_____	_____	_____
_____	_____	_____	_____
_____	_____	_____	_____
_____	_____	_____	_____
L_____	_____	S_____	_____
_____	_____	_____	_____
_____	_____	_____	_____
_____	_____	_____	_____
_____	_____		
_____	_____	TOTAL CALORIES/POINTS _____	

TUE

FOODS	CALORIES/POINTS	FOODS	CALORIES/POINTS
B_____	_____	D_____	_____
_____	_____	_____	_____
_____	_____	_____	_____
_____	_____	_____	_____
_____	_____	_____	_____
_____	_____	_____	_____
L_____	_____	S_____	_____
_____	_____	_____	_____
_____	_____	_____	_____
_____	_____	_____	_____
_____	_____		
_____	_____	TOTAL CALORIES/POINTS _____	

WED

FOODS	CALORIES/ POINTS	FOODS	CALORIES/ POINTS
B _____	_____	D _____	_____
_____	_____	_____	_____
_____	_____	_____	_____
_____	_____	_____	_____
_____	_____	_____	_____
_____	_____	_____	_____
L _____	_____	S _____	_____
_____	_____	_____	_____
_____	_____	_____	_____
_____	_____	_____	_____
_____	_____	TOTAL CALORIES/POINTS _____	

THU

FOODS	CALORIES/ POINTS	FOODS	CALORIES/ POINTS
B _____	_____	D _____	_____
_____	_____	_____	_____
_____	_____	_____	_____
_____	_____	_____	_____
_____	_____	_____	_____
_____	_____	_____	_____
L _____	_____	S _____	_____
_____	_____	_____	_____
_____	_____	_____	_____
_____	_____	_____	_____
_____	_____	TOTAL CALORIES/POINTS _____	

Calories/Points Tracker

FRI

FOODS	CALORIES/POINTS	FOODS	CALORIES/POINTS
B _____	_____	D _____	_____
_____	_____	_____	_____
_____	_____	_____	_____
_____	_____	_____	_____
_____	_____	_____	_____
_____	_____	_____	_____
L _____	_____	S _____	_____
_____	_____	_____	_____
_____	_____	_____	_____
_____	_____	_____	_____
_____	_____	TOTAL CALORIES/POINTS	_____
_____	_____		

SAT

FOODS	CALORIES/POINTS	FOODS	CALORIES/POINTS
B _____	_____	D _____	_____
_____	_____	_____	_____
_____	_____	_____	_____
_____	_____	_____	_____
_____	_____	_____	_____
_____	_____	_____	_____
L _____	_____	S _____	_____
_____	_____	_____	_____
_____	_____	_____	_____
_____	_____	_____	_____
_____	_____	TOTAL CALORIES/POINTS	_____

DATE ___ / ___ / ___ TO ___ / ___ / ___

FOODS	CALORIES/ POINTS	FOODS	CALORIES/ POINTS
B_____	___	D_____	___
_____	___	_____	___
_____	___	_____	___
_____	___	_____	___
_____	___	_____	___
_____	___	_____	___
L_____	___	S_____	___
_____	___	_____	___
_____	___	_____	___
_____	___	_____	___
_____	___		
_____	___	TOTAL CALORIES/POINTS ___	

—————— Exercise Tracker ——————

ACTIVITY	DISTANCE/ DURATION/INTENSITY	CALORIES BURNED
_____	_____	_____
_____	_____	_____
_____	_____	_____
_____	_____	_____
_____	_____	_____
_____	_____	_____
_____	_____	_____
_____	_____	_____

Weekly Meal Planner

Weekly Goals _____

_____

_____

_____

_____

superfood

APPLES

An apple a day . . . keeps you
healthy, always! Apples are a
perfectly compact, portable snack,
as well as a delicious add-in to
salads.

MON

TUE

WED

Calories/Points Tracker

DAILY GOAL

MON

FOODS	CALORIES/POINTS	FOODS	CALORIES/POINTS
B _____	___	D _____	___
_____	___	_____	___
_____	___	_____	___
_____	___	_____	___
_____	___	_____	___
_____	___	_____	___
L _____	___	S _____	___
_____	___	_____	___
_____	___	_____	___
_____	___	_____	___
_____	___		
_____	___	TOTAL CALORIES/POINTS ___	

TUE

FOODS	CALORIES/POINTS	FOODS	CALORIES/POINTS
B _____	___	D _____	___
_____	___	_____	___
_____	___	_____	___
_____	___	_____	___
_____	___	_____	___
_____	___	_____	___
L _____	___	S _____	___
_____	___	_____	___
_____	___	_____	___
_____	___	_____	___
_____	___		
_____	___	TOTAL CALORIES/POINTS ___	

DATE _____ / _____ / _____ TO _____ / _____ / _____

FOODS	CALORIES/POINTS	FOODS	CALORIES/POINTS
B _____	_____	D _____	_____
_____	_____	_____	_____
_____	_____	_____	_____
_____	_____	_____	_____
_____	_____	_____	_____
_____	_____	_____	_____
L _____	_____	S _____	_____
_____	_____	_____	_____
_____	_____	_____	_____
_____	_____	_____	_____
_____	_____		
_____	_____	TOTAL CALORIES/POINTS _____	

FOODS	CALORIES/POINTS	FOODS	CALORIES/POINTS
B _____	_____	D _____	_____
_____	_____	_____	_____
_____	_____	_____	_____
_____	_____	_____	_____
_____	_____	_____	_____
_____	_____	_____	_____
L _____	_____	S _____	_____
_____	_____	_____	_____
_____	_____	_____	_____
_____	_____	_____	_____
_____	_____		
_____	_____	TOTAL CALORIES/POINTS _____	

Calories/Points Tracker

DAILY GOAL

FRI

FOODS	CALORIES/POINTS	FOODS	CALORIES/POINTS
B_____ _____		D_____ _____	
_____ _____		_____ _____	
_____ _____		_____ _____	
_____ _____		_____ _____	
_____ _____		_____ _____	
_____ _____		_____ _____	
L_____ _____		S_____ _____	
_____ _____		_____ _____	
_____ _____		_____ _____	
_____ _____		_____ _____	
_____ _____			
_____ _____		TOTAL CALORIES/POINTS _____	

SAT

FOODS	CALORIES/POINTS	FOODS	CALORIES/POINTS
B_____ _____		D_____ _____	
_____ _____		_____ _____	
_____ _____		_____ _____	
_____ _____		_____ _____	
_____ _____		_____ _____	
_____ _____		_____ _____	
L_____ _____		S_____ _____	
_____ _____		_____ _____	
_____ _____		_____ _____	
_____ _____		_____ _____	
_____ _____			
_____ _____		TOTAL CALORIES/POINTS _____	

DATE _____ / _____ / _____ TO _____ / _____ / _____

FOODS	CALORIES/ POINTS	FOODS	CALORIES/ POINTS
B_____	____	D_____	____
_____	____	_____	____
_____	____	_____	____
_____	____	_____	____
_____	____	_____	____
_____	____	_____	____
L_____	____	S_____	____
_____	____	_____	____
_____	____	_____	____
_____	____	_____	____
_____	____		
_____	____	TOTAL CALORIES/POINTS ____	

Exercise Tracker

ACTIVITY	DISTANCE/ DURATION/INTENSITY	CALORIES BURNED
_____	_____	_____
_____	_____	_____
_____	_____	_____
_____	_____	_____
_____	_____	_____
_____	_____	_____
_____	_____	_____
_____	_____	_____

Weekly Meal Planner

Weekly Goals _____

_____

_____

_____

_____

MON

TUE

WED

Calories/Points Tracker

DAILY GOAL

MON

FOODS	CALORIES/ POINTS
B_____	_____
_____	_____
_____	_____
_____	_____
_____	_____
_____	_____
L_____	_____
_____	_____
_____	_____
_____	_____
_____	_____
_____	_____

FOODS	CALORIES/ POINTS
D_____	_____
_____	_____
_____	_____
_____	_____
_____	_____
S_____	_____
_____	_____
_____	_____
_____	_____
TOTAL CALORIES/POINTS	_____

TUE

FOODS	CALORIES/ POINTS
B_____	_____
_____	_____
_____	_____
_____	_____
_____	_____
_____	_____
L_____	_____
_____	_____
_____	_____
_____	_____
_____	_____
_____	_____

FOODS	CALORIES/ POINTS
D_____	_____
_____	_____
_____	_____
_____	_____
_____	_____
S_____	_____
_____	_____
_____	_____
_____	_____
TOTAL CALORIES/POINTS	_____

DATE ____/____/____ TO ____/____/____

FOODS	CALORIES/POINTS	FOODS	CALORIES/POINTS
B_____	_____	D_____	_____
_____	_____	_____	_____
_____	_____	_____	_____
_____	_____	_____	_____
_____	_____	_____	_____
_____	_____	_____	_____
L_____	_____	S_____	_____
_____	_____	_____	_____
_____	_____	_____	_____
_____	_____	_____	_____
_____	_____	TOTAL CALORIES/POINTS _____

FOODS	CALORIES/POINTS	FOODS	CALORIES/POINTS
B_____	_____	D_____	_____
_____	_____	_____	_____
_____	_____	_____	_____
_____	_____	_____	_____
_____	_____	_____	_____
_____	_____	_____	_____
L_____	_____	S_____	_____
_____	_____	_____	_____
_____	_____	_____	_____
_____	_____	_____	_____
_____	_____	TOTAL CALORIES/POINTS _____

Calories/Points Tracker

DAILY GOAL

FRI

FOODS	CALORIES/POINTS	FOODS	CALORIES/POINTS
B _____	____	D _____	____
_____	____	_____	____
_____	____	_____	____
_____	____	_____	____
_____	____	_____	____
_____	____	_____	____
L _____	____	S _____	____
_____	____	_____	____
_____	____	_____	____
_____	____	_____	____
_____	____	TOTAL CALORIES/POINTS ____
_____	____		

SAT

FOODS	CALORIES/POINTS	FOODS	CALORIES/POINTS
B _____	____	D _____	____
_____	____	_____	____
_____	____	_____	____
_____	____	_____	____
_____	____	_____	____
_____	____	_____	____
L _____	____	S _____	____
_____	____	_____	____
_____	____	_____	____
_____	____	_____	____
_____	____	TOTAL CALORIES/POINTS ____
_____	____		

DATE ___ / ___ / ___ TO ___ / ___ / ___

FOODS	CALORIES/POINTS	FOODS	CALORIES/POINTS
B_____	___	D_____	___
_____	___	_____	___
_____	___	_____	___
_____	___	_____	___
_____	___	_____	___
_____	___	_____	___
L_____	___	S_____	___
_____	___	_____	___
_____	___	_____	___
_____	___	_____	___
_____	___		
_____	___	TOTAL CALORIES/POINTS ___	

──────────── Exercise Tracker ────────────

ACTIVITY	DISTANCE/DURATION/INTENSITY	CALORIES BURNED
_____	_____	_____
_____	_____	_____
_____	_____	_____
_____	_____	_____
_____	_____	_____
_____	_____	_____
_____	_____	_____
_____	_____	_____

Sweet Potato, Kale, and Chicken Soup

SERVES 6

2 chicken breasts, on the bone, skin removed (26 ounces) or 16-ounce boneless

1 teaspoon seasoning salt (such as adobo)

½ teaspoon olive oil

1 large onion, chopped

2 celery stalks, chopped

3 garlic cloves, chopped

½ teaspoon dried oregano

½ teaspoon dried thyme

½ teaspoon ground cumin

6 cups reduced-sodium chicken broth

1 fresh jalapeño, sliced in half lengthwise

¼ cup chopped fresh cilantro

1 large sweet potato, peeled and cut into 1-inch cubes

3 cups kale, stemmed and roughly chopped

SERVING SIZE	1½ cups
CALORIES	191
FAT	3 g
CHOLESTEROL	55 mg
CARBOHYDRATE	10 g
FIBER	3.5 g
PROTEIN	21.5 g
SUGAR	2 g
SODIUM	880 mg

Season the chicken with the seasoning salt and set aside.

Heat a large nonstick pot or Dutch oven over medium-low heat. Add the oil, onions, and celery, and cook, stirring, until soft and golden, 8 to 10 minutes. Add the garlic, oregano, thyme, and cumin, and cook, stirring, 2 to 3 minutes. Add the chicken, chicken broth, jalapeño, and cilantro. Cover and cook 20 minutes. Add the sweet potato and kale and cook until the sweet potatoes are tender and the chicken is cooked, 25 to 30 minutes.

Remove the chicken from the pot, shred the meat, and discard the bones. Return the chicken to the pot, discard the jalapeño, and serve.

Weekly Meal Planner

Weekly Goals _____

_____

_____

_____

_____

"If you can dream
it, you can do it."

WALT DISNEY

MON

TUE

WED

THU

FRI

SAT

SUN

Calories/Points Tracker

MON

FOODS	CALORIES/ POINTS
B_____	_____
_____	_____
_____	_____
_____	_____
_____	_____
_____	_____
L_____	_____
_____	_____
_____	_____
_____	_____
_____	_____
_____	_____

FOODS	CALORIES/ POINTS
D_____	_____
_____	_____
_____	_____
_____	_____
_____	_____
S_____	_____
_____	_____
_____	_____
_____	_____
TOTAL CALORIES/POINTS	_____

TUE

FOODS	CALORIES/ POINTS
B_____	_____
_____	_____
_____	_____
_____	_____
_____	_____
_____	_____
L_____	_____
_____	_____
_____	_____
_____	_____
_____	_____
_____	_____

FOODS	CALORIES/ POINTS
D_____	_____
_____	_____
_____	_____
_____	_____
_____	_____
S_____	_____
_____	_____
_____	_____
_____	_____
TOTAL CALORIES/POINTS	_____

DATE ____ / ____ / ____ TO ____ / ____ / ____

FOODS	CALORIES/ POINTS	FOODS	CALORIES/ POINTS
B_____ ____		D_____ ____	
_____ ____		_____ ____	
_____ ____		_____ ____	
_____ ____		_____ ____	
_____ ____		_____ ____	
_____ ____		_____ ____	
L_____ ____		S_____ ____	
_____ ____		_____ ____	
_____ ____		_____ ____	
_____ ____		_____ ____	
_____ ____			
_____ ____		TOTAL CALORIES/POINTS ____	

FOODS	CALORIES/ POINTS	FOODS	CALORIES/ POINTS
B_____ ____		D_____ ____	
_____ ____		_____ ____	
_____ ____		_____ ____	
_____ ____		_____ ____	
_____ ____		_____ ____	
_____ ____		_____ ____	
L_____ ____		S_____ ____	
_____ ____		_____ ____	
_____ ____		_____ ____	
_____ ____		_____ ____	
_____ ____			
_____ ____		TOTAL CALORIES/POINTS ____	

Calories/Points Tracker

FRI

FOODS   CALORIES/POINTS

B _____ _____

_____ _____

_____ _____

_____ _____

_____ _____

_____ _____

L _____ _____

_____ _____

_____ _____

_____ _____

_____ _____

FOODS   CALORIES/POINTS

D _____ _____

_____ _____

_____ _____

_____ _____

_____ _____

S _____ _____

_____ _____

_____ _____

_____ _____

TOTAL CALORIES/POINTS _____

SAT

FOODS   CALORIES/POINTS

B _____ _____

_____ _____

_____ _____

_____ _____

_____ _____

_____ _____

L _____ _____

_____ _____

_____ _____

_____ _____

_____ _____

FOODS   CALORIES/POINTS

D _____ _____

_____ _____

_____ _____

_____ _____

_____ _____

S _____ _____

_____ _____

_____ _____

_____ _____

TOTAL CALORIES/POINTS _____

DATE ___ / ___ / ___ TO ___ / ___ / ___

FOODS	CALORIES/ POINTS	FOODS	CALORIES/ POINTS
B _____ ___		D _____ ___	
_____ ___		_____ ___	
_____ ___		_____ ___	
_____ ___		_____ ___	
_____ ___		_____ ___	
_____ ___		_____ ___	
L _____ ___		S _____ ___	
_____ ___		_____ ___	
_____ ___		_____ ___	
_____ ___		_____ ___	
_____ ___			
_____ ___		TOTAL CALORIES/POINTS ___	

—————————— Exercise Tracker ——————————

ACTIVITY	DISTANCE/ DURATION/INTENSITY	CALORIES BURNED
_____	_____	_____
_____	_____	_____
_____	_____	_____
_____	_____	_____
_____	_____	_____
_____	_____	_____
_____	_____	_____
_____	_____	_____

Weekly Meal Planner

Weekly Goals _____

_____

_____

_____

_____

MON

TUE

WED

Calories/Points Tracker

MON

FOODS	CALORIES/POINTS
B_____	_____
_____	_____
_____	_____
_____	_____
_____	_____
_____	_____
L_____	_____
_____	_____
_____	_____
_____	_____
_____	_____
_____	_____

FOODS	CALORIES/POINTS
D_____	_____
_____	_____
_____	_____
_____	_____
_____	_____
S_____	_____
_____	_____
_____	_____
_____	_____
TOTAL CALORIES/POINTS	_____

TUE

FOODS	CALORIES/POINTS
B_____	_____
_____	_____
_____	_____
_____	_____
_____	_____
_____	_____
L_____	_____
_____	_____
_____	_____
_____	_____
_____	_____
_____	_____

FOODS	CALORIES/POINTS
D_____	_____
_____	_____
_____	_____
_____	_____
_____	_____
S_____	_____
_____	_____
_____	_____
_____	_____
TOTAL CALORIES/POINTS	_____

FOODS	CALORIES/ POINTS	FOODS	CALORIES/ POINTS
B _____	___	D _____	___
_____	___	_____	___
_____	___	_____	___
_____	___	_____	___
_____	___	_____	___
_____	___	_____	___
L _____	___	S _____	___
_____	___	_____	___
_____	___	_____	___
_____	___	_____	___
_____	___	TOTAL CALORIES/POINTS ___	
_____	___		

FOODS	CALORIES/ POINTS	FOODS	CALORIES/ POINTS
B _____	___	D _____	___
_____	___	_____	___
_____	___	_____	___
_____	___	_____	___
_____	___	_____	___
_____	___	_____	___
L _____	___	S _____	___
_____	___	_____	___
_____	___	_____	___
_____	___	_____	___
_____	___	TOTAL CALORIES/POINTS ___	
_____	___		

Calories/Points Tracker

DAILY GOAL _____

FRI

FOODS	CALORIES/ POINTS
B _____	_____
_____	_____
_____	_____
_____	_____
_____	_____
_____	_____
L _____	_____
_____	_____
_____	_____
_____	_____
_____	_____
_____	_____

FOODS	CALORIES/ POINTS
D _____	_____
_____	_____
_____	_____
_____	_____
_____	_____
S _____	_____
_____	_____
_____	_____
_____	_____

TOTAL CALORIES/POINTS _____

SAT

FOODS	CALORIES/ POINTS
B _____	_____
_____	_____
_____	_____
_____	_____
_____	_____
_____	_____
L _____	_____
_____	_____
_____	_____
_____	_____
_____	_____
_____	_____

FOODS	CALORIES/ POINTS
D _____	_____
_____	_____
_____	_____
_____	_____
_____	_____
S _____	_____
_____	_____
_____	_____
_____	_____

TOTAL CALORIES/POINTS _____

DATE ____ / ____ / ____ TO ____ / ____ / ____

FOODS	CALORIES/ POINTS	FOODS	CALORIES/ POINTS
B_____	_____	D_____	_____
_____	_____	_____	_____
_____	_____	_____	_____
_____	_____	_____	_____
_____	_____	_____	_____
_____	_____	_____	_____
L_____	_____	S_____	_____
_____	_____	_____	_____
_____	_____	_____	_____
_____	_____	_____	_____
_____	_____	TOTAL CALORIES/POINTS _____
_____	_____		

―――――――――――――― Exercise Tracker ――――――――――――――

ACTIVITY	DISTANCE/ DURATION/INTENSITY	CALORIES BURNED
_____	_____	_____
_____	_____	_____
_____	_____	_____
_____	_____	_____
_____	_____	_____
_____	_____	_____
_____	_____	_____

Weekly Meal Planner

Weekly Goals _____

_____

_____

_____

_____

> "The secret of getting ahead is getting started."
>
> MARK TWAIN

MON

_____

_____

_____

_____

TUE

_____

_____

_____

_____

WED

_____

_____

_____

_____

Calories/Points Tracker

DAILY GOAL _____

MON

FOODS	CALORIES/POINTS	FOODS	CALORIES/POINTS
B_____	____	D_____	____
_____	____	_____	____
_____	____	_____	____
_____	____	_____	____
_____	____	_____	____
_____	____	_____	____
L_____	____	S_____	____
_____	____	_____	____
_____	____	_____	____
_____	____	_____	____
_____	____	TOTAL CALORIES/POINTS ____	

TUE

FOODS	CALORIES/POINTS	FOODS	CALORIES/POINTS
B_____	____	D_____	____
_____	____	_____	____
_____	____	_____	____
_____	____	_____	____
_____	____	_____	____
_____	____	_____	____
L_____	____	S_____	____
_____	____	_____	____
_____	____	_____	____
_____	____	_____	____
_____	____	TOTAL CALORIES/POINTS ____	

DATE ___ / ___ / ___ TO ___ / ___ / ___

FOODS	CALORIES/POINTS	FOODS	CALORIES/POINTS
B _____ _____		D _____ _____	
_____ _____		_____ _____	
_____ _____		_____ _____	
_____ _____		_____ _____	
_____ _____		_____ _____	
_____ _____		_____ _____	
L _____ _____		S _____ _____	
_____ _____		_____ _____	
_____ _____		_____ _____	
_____ _____		_____ _____	
_____ _____		TOTAL CALORIES/POINTS _____	

FOODS	CALORIES/POINTS	FOODS	CALORIES/POINTS
B _____ _____		D _____ _____	
_____ _____		_____ _____	
_____ _____		_____ _____	
_____ _____		_____ _____	
_____ _____		_____ _____	
_____ _____		_____ _____	
L _____ _____		S _____ _____	
_____ _____		_____ _____	
_____ _____		_____ _____	
_____ _____		_____ _____	
_____ _____		TOTAL CALORIES/POINTS _____	

Calories/Points Tracker

FRI

FOODS	CALORIES/POINTS	FOODS	CALORIES/POINTS
B _____	_____	D _____	_____
_____	_____	_____	_____
_____	_____	_____	_____
_____	_____	_____	_____
_____	_____	_____	_____
_____	_____	_____	_____
L _____	_____	S _____	_____
_____	_____	_____	_____
_____	_____	_____	_____
_____	_____	_____	_____
_____	_____	
_____	_____	TOTAL CALORIES/POINTS _____

SAT

FOODS	CALORIES/POINTS	FOODS	CALORIES/POINTS
B _____	_____	D _____	_____
_____	_____	_____	_____
_____	_____	_____	_____
_____	_____	_____	_____
_____	_____	_____	_____
_____	_____	_____	_____
L _____	_____	S _____	_____
_____	_____	_____	_____
_____	_____	_____	_____
_____	_____	_____	_____
_____	_____	
_____	_____	TOTAL CALORIES/POINTS _____

DATE _____ / _____ / _____ TO _____ / _____ / _____

FOODS	CALORIES/POINTS	FOODS	CALORIES/POINTS
B_____ _____		D_____ _____	
_____ _____		_____ _____	
_____ _____		_____ _____	
_____ _____		_____ _____	
_____ _____		_____ _____	
_____ _____		_____ _____	
L_____ _____		S_____ _____	
_____ _____		_____ _____	
_____ _____		_____ _____	
_____ _____		_____ _____	
_____ _____			
_____ _____		TOTAL CALORIES/POINTS _____	

—————————————— Exercise Tracker ——————————————

ACTIVITY	DISTANCE/DURATION/INTENSITY	CALORIES BURNED
_____	_____	_____
_____	_____	_____
_____	_____	_____
_____	_____	_____
_____	_____	_____
_____	_____	_____
_____	_____	_____

Easy Pumpkin-Spice Granola

MAKES 3 ⅔ CUPS; SERVES 11

¼ cup uncooked quinoa

1½ cups rolled oats*

¼ cup ground flaxseeds

¼ cup pepitas (or other seed)

¼ cup chopped pecans

½ cup dried cranberries

¼ cup real maple syrup or honey

¼ cup pumpkin puree

1 teaspoon coconut oil or canola oil

½ teaspoon vanilla extract

1 teaspoon pumpkin spice (or more to taste)

¼ teaspoon ground cinnamon

Pinch of kosher salt

SERVING SIZE	½ cup
CALORIES	128
FAT	4.5 g
CHOLESTEROL	0 mg
CARBOHYDRATE	20 g
FIBER	3 g
PROTEIN	3 g
SUGAR	7 g
SODIUM	16 mg

Preheat the oven to 325°F.

Rinse the quinoa, drain, and dry well on paper towels. Spread the quinoa and oats out on a parchment paper-lined baking sheet. Toast in the oven, stirring once, for 10 minutes.

Transfer the quinoa and oats to a medium bowl and add the ground flaxseeds, pepitas, pecans, and dried cranberries.

Reduce the oven to 300°F.

In a second medium bowl, combine the maple syrup, pumpkin puree, oil, vanilla extract, pumpkin spice, cinnamon, and salt. Pour the mixture over the oats and stir well. Spread back onto the baking sheet.

Bake until golden, 20 minutes.

Use gluten-free oats for gluten allergies.

Weekly Meal Planner

Weekly Goals _____

_____

_____

_____

_____

superfood

DARK CHOCOLATE

Here's your license to eat some chocolate! Just a small square a day will give your body a dose of healthy antioxidants.

MON

TUE

WED

Calories/Points Tracker

MON

FOODS	CALORIES/ POINTS
B_____	_____
_____	_____
_____	_____
_____	_____
_____	_____
_____	_____
L_____	_____
_____	_____
_____	_____
_____	_____
_____	_____
_____	_____

FOODS	CALORIES/ POINTS
D_____	_____
_____	_____
_____	_____
_____	_____
_____	_____
S_____	_____
_____	_____
_____	_____
_____	_____

TOTAL CALORIES/POINTS _____

TUE

FOODS	CALORIES/ POINTS
B_____	_____
_____	_____
_____	_____
_____	_____
_____	_____
_____	_____
L_____	_____
_____	_____
_____	_____
_____	_____
_____	_____
_____	_____

FOODS	CALORIES/ POINTS
D_____	_____
_____	_____
_____	_____
_____	_____
_____	_____
S_____	_____
_____	_____
_____	_____
_____	_____

TOTAL CALORIES/POINTS _____

DATE ___ / ___ / ___ TO ___ / ___ / ___

FOODS	CALORIES/ POINTS	FOODS	CALORIES/ POINTS
B_____ ___		D_____ ___	
_____ ___		_____ ___	
_____ ___		_____ ___	
_____ ___		_____ ___	
_____ ___		_____ ___	
_____ ___		_____ ___	
L_____ ___		S_____ ___	
_____ ___		_____ ___	
_____ ___		_____ ___	
_____ ___		_____ ___	
_____ ___		_____ ___	
_____ ___		TOTAL CALORIES/POINTS ___	

FOODS	CALORIES/ POINTS	FOODS	CALORIES/ POINTS
B_____ ___		D_____ ___	
_____ ___		_____ ___	
_____ ___		_____ ___	
_____ ___		_____ ___	
_____ ___		_____ ___	
_____ ___		_____ ___	
L_____ ___		S_____ ___	
_____ ___		_____ ___	
_____ ___		_____ ___	
_____ ___		_____ ___	
_____ ___		_____ ___	
_____ ___		TOTAL CALORIES/POINTS ___	

Calories/Points Tracker

DAILY GOAL

FRI

FOODS	CALORIES/POINTS	FOODS	CALORIES/POINTS
B_____	_____	D_____	_____
_____	_____	_____	_____
_____	_____	_____	_____
_____	_____	_____	_____
_____	_____	_____	_____
_____	_____	_____	_____
L_____	_____	S_____	_____
_____	_____	_____	_____
_____	_____	_____	_____
_____	_____	_____	_____
_____	_____	_____	_____
_____	_____	

TOTAL CALORIES/POINTS _____

SAT

FOODS	CALORIES/POINTS	FOODS	CALORIES/POINTS
B_____	_____	D_____	_____
_____	_____	_____	_____
_____	_____	_____	_____
_____	_____	_____	_____
_____	_____	_____	_____
_____	_____	_____	_____
L_____	_____	S_____	_____
_____	_____	_____	_____
_____	_____	_____	_____
_____	_____	_____	_____
_____	_____	_____	_____
_____	_____	

TOTAL CALORIES/POINTS _____

DATE ___ / ___ / ___ TO ___ / ___ / ___

FOODS	CALORIES/POINTS	FOODS	CALORIES/POINTS
B_____	_____	D_____	_____
_____	_____	_____	_____
_____	_____	_____	_____
_____	_____	_____	_____
_____	_____	_____	_____
_____	_____	_____	_____
L_____	_____	S_____	_____
_____	_____	_____	_____
_____	_____	_____	_____
_____	_____	_____	_____
_____	_____	TOTAL CALORIES/POINTS _____
_____	_____		

—————————————— Exercise Tracker ——————————————

ACTIVITY	DISTANCE/DURATION/INTENSITY	CALORIES BURNED
_____	_____	_____
_____	_____	_____
_____	_____	_____
_____	_____	_____
_____	_____	_____
_____	_____	_____
_____	_____	_____
_____	_____	_____

Weekly Meal Planner

Weekly Goals _____

_____

_____

_____

_____

> "It's not the years in your life that count. It's the life in your years."
>
> **ABRAHAM LINCOLN**

MON

TUE

WED

THU

FRI

SAT

SUN

Calories/Points Tracker

DAILY GOAL

MON

FOODS	CALORIES/POINTS
B _____	_____
_____	_____
_____	_____
_____	_____
_____	_____
L _____	_____
_____	_____
_____	_____
_____	_____
_____	_____

FOODS	CALORIES/POINTS
D _____	_____
_____	_____
_____	_____
_____	_____
_____	_____
S _____	_____
_____	_____
_____	_____
_____	_____

TOTAL CALORIES/POINTS _____

TUE

FOODS	CALORIES/POINTS
B _____	_____
_____	_____
_____	_____
_____	_____
_____	_____
L _____	_____
_____	_____
_____	_____
_____	_____
_____	_____

FOODS	CALORIES/POINTS
D _____	_____
_____	_____
_____	_____
_____	_____
_____	_____
S _____	_____
_____	_____
_____	_____
_____	_____

TOTAL CALORIES/POINTS _____

DATE ____ / ____ / ____ TO ____ / ____ / ____

FOODS	CALORIES/ POINTS	FOODS	CALORIES/ POINTS
B_____ _____		D_____ _____	
_____ _____		_____ _____	
_____ _____		_____ _____	
_____ _____		_____ _____	
_____ _____		_____ _____	
_____ _____		_____ _____	
L_____ _____		S_____ _____	
_____ _____		_____ _____	
_____ _____		_____ _____	
_____ _____		_____ _____	
_____ _____		_____ _____	
_____ _____		TOTAL CALORIES/POINTS _____	

FOODS	CALORIES/ POINTS	FOODS	CALORIES/ POINTS
B_____ _____		D_____ _____	
_____ _____		_____ _____	
_____ _____		_____ _____	
_____ _____		_____ _____	
_____ _____		_____ _____	
_____ _____		_____ _____	
L_____ _____		S_____ _____	
_____ _____		_____ _____	
_____ _____		_____ _____	
_____ _____		_____ _____	
_____ _____		_____ _____	
_____ _____		TOTAL CALORIES/POINTS _____	

Calories/Points Tracker

DAILY GOAL _____

FRI

FOODS	CALORIES/ POINTS	FOODS	CALORIES/ POINTS
B_____	_____	D_____	_____
_____	_____	_____	_____
_____	_____	_____	_____
_____	_____	_____	_____
_____	_____	_____	_____
L_____	_____	S_____	_____
_____	_____	_____	_____
_____	_____	_____	_____
_____	_____	_____	_____
_____	_____	TOTAL CALORIES/POINTS _____

SAT

FOODS	CALORIES/ POINTS	FOODS	CALORIES/ POINTS
B_____	_____	D_____	_____
_____	_____	_____	_____
_____	_____	_____	_____
_____	_____	_____	_____
_____	_____	_____	_____
L_____	_____	S_____	_____
_____	_____	_____	_____
_____	_____	_____	_____
_____	_____	_____	_____
_____	_____	TOTAL CALORIES/POINTS _____

DATE _____ / _____ / _____ TO _____ / _____ / _____

FOODS	CALORIES/ POINTS	FOODS	CALORIES/ POINTS
B_____	_____	D_____	_____
_____	_____	_____	_____
_____	_____	_____	_____
_____	_____	_____	_____
_____	_____	_____	_____
_____	_____	_____	_____
L_____	_____	S_____	_____
_____	_____	_____	_____
_____	_____	_____	_____
_____	_____	_____	_____
_____	_____		
_____	_____	TOTAL CALORIES/POINTS _____	

—————— Exercise Tracker ——————

ACTIVITY	DISTANCE/ DURATION/INTENSITY	CALORIES BURNED
_____	_____	_____
_____	_____	_____
_____	_____	_____
_____	_____	_____
_____	_____	_____
_____	_____	_____
_____	_____	_____

Weekly Meal Planner

Weekly Goals _____

_____

_____

_____

_____

> "Change your
> thoughts and
> you change your
> world."
>
> **NORMAN VINCENT PEALE**

MON

TUE

WED

Calories/Points Tracker

MON

FOODS	CALORIES/POINTS	FOODS	CALORIES/POINTS
B		D	
L		S	
		TOTAL CALORIES/POINTS	

TUE

FOODS	CALORIES/POINTS	FOODS	CALORIES/POINTS
B		D	
L		S	
		TOTAL CALORIES/POINTS	

DATE ___ / ___ / ___ TO ___ / ___ / ___

FOODS	CALORIES/POINTS	FOODS	CALORIES/POINTS
B _____ ____		D _____ ____	
_____ ____		_____ ____	
_____ ____		_____ ____	
_____ ____		_____ ____	
_____ ____		_____ ____	
_____ ____		_____ ____	
L _____ ____		S _____ ____	
_____ ____		_____ ____	
_____ ____		_____ ____	
_____ ____		_____ ____	
_____ ____		TOTAL CALORIES/POINTS ____	

FOODS	CALORIES/POINTS	FOODS	CALORIES/POINTS
B _____ ____		D _____ ____	
_____ ____		_____ ____	
_____ ____		_____ ____	
_____ ____		_____ ____	
_____ ____		_____ ____	
_____ ____		_____ ____	
L _____ ____		S _____ ____	
_____ ____		_____ ____	
_____ ____		_____ ____	
_____ ____		_____ ____	
_____ ____		TOTAL CALORIES/POINTS ____	

Calories/Points Tracker

DAILY GOAL

FRI

FOODS	CALORIES/ POINTS	FOODS	CALORIES/ POINTS
B _____	_____	D _____	_____
_____	_____	_____	_____
_____	_____	_____	_____
_____	_____	_____	_____
_____	_____	_____	_____
_____	_____	_____	_____
L _____	_____	S _____	_____
_____	_____	_____	_____
_____	_____	_____	_____
_____	_____	_____	_____
_____	_____		
_____	_____	TOTAL CALORIES/POINTS _____	

SAT

FOODS	CALORIES/ POINTS	FOODS	CALORIES/ POINTS
B _____	_____	D _____	_____
_____	_____	_____	_____
_____	_____	_____	_____
_____	_____	_____	_____
_____	_____	_____	_____
_____	_____	_____	_____
L _____	_____	S _____	_____
_____	_____	_____	_____
_____	_____	_____	_____
_____	_____	_____	_____
_____	_____		
_____	_____	TOTAL CALORIES/POINTS _____	

DATE ___/___/___ TO ___/___/___

FOODS	CALORIES/POINTS	FOODS	CALORIES/POINTS
B _____	___	D _____	___
_____	___	_____	___
_____	___	_____	___
_____	___	_____	___
_____	___	_____	___
_____	___	_____	___
L _____	___	S _____	___
_____	___	_____	___
_____	___	_____	___
_____	___	_____	___
_____	___		
_____	___	TOTAL CALORIES/POINTS ___	

——————————— Exercise Tracker ———————————

ACTIVITY	DISTANCE/DURATION/INTENSITY	CALORIES BURNED
_____	_____	_____
_____	_____	_____
_____	_____	_____
_____	_____	_____
_____	_____	_____
_____	_____	_____
_____	_____	_____
_____	_____	_____

Dark Chocolate Cranberry Pistachio-Bark

SERVES 14

7 ounces dark chocolate
(calculations based on Hershey's
Special Dark)

4.5 ounces shelled pistachios,
coarsely chopped

2.5 ounces dried cranberries,
coarsely chopped

SERVING SIZE	1 ounce (a roughly 3½ x 3½-inch piece
CALORIES	126.6
FAT	8.1 g
CHOLESTEROL	2 mg
CARBOHYDRATE	15.3 g
FIBER	2.1 g
PROTEIN	2.6 g
SUGAR	10.7 g
SODIUM	1.1 mg

Place the chocolate in a microwave-safe measuring cup. Microwave on High for 1 minute, stirring every 15 seconds, or until the chocolate melts. Pour the chocolate into a bowl and stir in the pistachios and dried cranberries. Spread the mixture evenly on a jelly-roll pan lined with foil. Freeze for 1 hour.

Remove from the freezer, break the bark into pieces, and enjoy. The bark will keep in an airtight container in the fridge or a cool room for up to 3 weeks.

Matcha Green Tea Shots

MAKES 2; SERVES 2

1 cup sweetened vanilla almond milk
(I like Almond Breeze)

2 teaspoons Matcha powder

SERVING SIZE	2 shots
CALORIES	50
FAT	2 g
CHOLESTEROL	0 mg
CARBOHYDRATE	9 g
FIBER	1 g
PROTEIN	1 g
SUGAR	7.5 g
SODIUM	76 mg

Combine the almond milk and Matcha powder in a martini shaker. Shake really well to dissolve the powder. Pour into four shot glasses and serve, two per person.

Weekly Meal Planner

Weekly Goals _____

_____ _____

_____

_____

_____

superfood

GREEN TEA

Try swapping out a cup (or two) of coffee each day with green tea. You'll get the same caffeine pick-me-up, with more antioxidants for your body.

MON

TUE

WED

Calories/Points Tracker

DAILY GOAL

MON

FOODS	CALORIES/POINTS	FOODS	CALORIES/POINTS
B_____	_____	D_____	_____
_____	_____	_____	_____
_____	_____	_____	_____
_____	_____	_____	_____
_____	_____	_____	_____
_____	_____	_____	_____
L_____	_____	S_____	_____
_____	_____	_____	_____
_____	_____	_____	_____
_____	_____	_____	_____
_____	_____		
_____	_____	TOTAL CALORIES/POINTS _____	

TUE

FOODS	CALORIES/POINTS	FOODS	CALORIES/POINTS
B_____	_____	D_____	_____
_____	_____	_____	_____
_____	_____	_____	_____
_____	_____	_____	_____
_____	_____	_____	_____
_____	_____	_____	_____
L_____	_____	S_____	_____
_____	_____	_____	_____
_____	_____	_____	_____
_____	_____	_____	_____
_____	_____		
_____	_____	TOTAL CALORIES/POINTS _____	

DATE ___/___/___ TO ___/___/___

FOODS	CALORIES/POINTS	FOODS	CALORIES/POINTS
B_____	_____	D_____	_____
_____	_____	_____	_____
_____	_____	_____	_____
_____	_____	_____	_____
_____	_____	_____	_____
_____	_____	_____	_____
L_____	_____	S_____	_____
_____	_____	_____	_____
_____	_____	_____	_____
_____	_____	_____	_____
_____	_____		
_____	_____	TOTAL CALORIES/POINTS _____	

FOODS	CALORIES/POINTS	FOODS	CALORIES/POINTS
B_____	_____	D_____	_____
_____	_____	_____	_____
_____	_____	_____	_____
_____	_____	_____	_____
_____	_____	_____	_____
_____	_____	_____	_____
L_____	_____	S_____	_____
_____	_____	_____	_____
_____	_____	_____	_____
_____	_____	_____	_____
_____	_____		
_____	_____	TOTAL CALORIES/POINTS _____	

Calories/Points Tracker

DAILY GOAL

FRI

FOODS	CALORIES/POINTS
B_____	_____
_____	_____
_____	_____
_____	_____
_____	_____
_____	_____
L_____	_____
_____	_____
_____	_____
_____	_____
_____	_____
_____	_____

FOODS	CALORIES/POINTS
D_____	_____
_____	_____
_____	_____
_____	_____
_____	_____
_____	_____
S_____	_____
_____	_____
_____	_____
_____	_____
TOTAL CALORIES/POINTS	_____

SAT

FOODS	CALORIES/POINTS
B_____	_____
_____	_____
_____	_____
_____	_____
_____	_____
_____	_____
L_____	_____
_____	_____
_____	_____
_____	_____
_____	_____
_____	_____

FOODS	CALORIES/POINTS
D_____	_____
_____	_____
_____	_____
_____	_____
_____	_____
_____	_____
S_____	_____
_____	_____
_____	_____
_____	_____
TOTAL CALORIES/POINTS	_____

SUN

DATE ___/___/___ TO ___/___/___

FOODS	CALORIES/ POINTS	FOODS	CALORIES/ POINTS
B_____	___	D_____	___
_____	___	_____	___
_____	___	_____	___
_____	___	_____	___
_____	___	_____	___
_____	___	_____	___
L_____	___	S_____	___
_____	___	_____	___
_____	___	_____	___
_____	___	_____	___
_____	___		
_____	___	TOTAL CALORIES/POINTS ___	

——————————— Exercise Tracker ———————————

ACTIVITY	DISTANCE/ DURATION/INTENSITY	CALORIES BURNED
_____	_____	_____
_____	_____	_____
_____	_____	_____
_____	_____	_____
_____	_____	_____
_____	_____	_____
_____	_____	_____
_____	_____	_____

Weekly Meal Planner

Weekly Goals _____

_____

_____

_____

_____

MON

_____

_____

_____

_____

TUE

_____

_____

_____

_____

WED

_____

_____

_____

_____

THU

FRI

SAT

SUN

Calories/Points Tracker

DAILY GOAL _____

MON

FOODS	CALORIES/POINTS
B _____	_____
_____	_____
_____	_____
_____	_____
_____	_____
_____	_____
L _____	_____
_____	_____
_____	_____
_____	_____
_____	_____
_____	_____

FOODS	CALORIES/POINTS
D _____	_____
_____	_____
_____	_____
_____	_____
_____	_____
_____	_____
S _____	_____
_____	_____
_____	_____
_____	_____

TOTAL CALORIES/POINTS _____

TUE

FOODS	CALORIES/POINTS
B _____	_____
_____	_____
_____	_____
_____	_____
_____	_____
_____	_____
L _____	_____
_____	_____
_____	_____
_____	_____
_____	_____
_____	_____

FOODS	CALORIES/POINTS
D _____	_____
_____	_____
_____	_____
_____	_____
_____	_____
_____	_____
S _____	_____
_____	_____
_____	_____
_____	_____

TOTAL CALORIES/POINTS _____

DATE ___ / ___ / ___ TO ___ / ___ / ___

FOODS	CALORIES/ POINTS	FOODS	CALORIES/ POINTS
B_____ ____		D_____ ____	
_____ ____		_____ ____	
_____ ____		_____ ____	
_____ ____		_____ ____	
_____ ____		_____ ____	
_____ ____		_____ ____	
L_____ ____		S_____ ____	
_____ ____		_____ ____	
_____ ____		_____ ____	
_____ ____		_____ ____	
_____ ____		_____ ____	
_____ ____		TOTAL CALORIES/POINTS ____	

FOODS	CALORIES/ POINTS	FOODS	CALORIES/ POINTS
B_____ ____		D_____ ____	
_____ ____		_____ ____	
_____ ____		_____ ____	
_____ ____		_____ ____	
_____ ____		_____ ____	
_____ ____		_____ ____	
L_____ ____		S_____ ____	
_____ ____		_____ ____	
_____ ____		_____ ____	
_____ ____		_____ ____	
_____ ____		TOTAL CALORIES/POINTS ____	

Calories/Points Tracker

DAILY GOAL

FOODS	CALORIES/POINTS	FOODS	CALORIES/POINTS

FRI

B _____ _____

_____ _____

_____ _____

_____ _____

_____ _____

_____ _____

L _____ _____

_____ _____

_____ _____

_____ _____

_____ _____

_____ _____

D _____ _____

_____ _____

_____ _____

_____ _____

_____ _____

S _____ _____

_____ _____

_____ _____

_____ _____

TOTAL CALORIES/POINTS _____

FOODS	CALORIES/POINTS	FOODS	CALORIES/POINTS

SAT

B _____ _____

_____ _____

_____ _____

_____ _____

_____ _____

_____ _____

L _____ _____

_____ _____

_____ _____

_____ _____

_____ _____

_____ _____

D _____ _____

_____ _____

_____ _____

_____ _____

_____ _____

S _____ _____

_____ _____

_____ _____

_____ _____

TOTAL CALORIES/POINTS _____

DATE _____ / _____ / _____ TO _____ / _____ / _____

FOODS	CALORIES/ POINTS	FOODS	CALORIES/ POINTS
B _____	_____	D _____	_____
_____	_____	_____	_____
_____	_____	_____	_____
_____	_____	_____	_____
_____	_____	_____	_____
_____	_____	_____	_____
L _____	_____	S _____	_____
_____	_____	_____	_____
_____	_____	_____	_____
_____	_____	_____	_____
_____	_____		
_____	_____	TOTAL CALORIES/POINTS _____	

—————— Exercise Tracker ——————

ACTIVITY	DISTANCE/ DURATION/INTENSITY	CALORIES BURNED
_____	_____	_____
_____	_____	_____
_____	_____	_____
_____	_____	_____
_____	_____	_____
_____	_____	_____
_____	_____	_____
_____	_____	_____

Weekly Meal Planner

Weekly Goals _____

_____

_____

_____

_____

superfood

GARLIC

Though the taste may be strong to some, garlic is one of my favorite foods. I love its pungency in everything from a bright vinaigrette to roasted vegetables and meats.

MON

TUE

WED

Calories/Points Tracker

DAILY GOAL

MON

FOODS	CALORIES/ POINTS	FOODS	CALORIES/ POINTS
B_____	_____	D_____	_____
_____	_____	_____	_____
_____	_____	_____	_____
_____	_____	_____	_____
_____	_____	_____	_____
_____	_____	_____	_____
L_____	_____	S_____	_____
_____	_____	_____	_____
_____	_____	_____	_____
_____	_____	_____	_____
_____	_____	TOTAL CALORIES/POINTS _____	

TUE

FOODS	CALORIES/ POINTS	FOODS	CALORIES/ POINTS
B_____	_____	D_____	_____
_____	_____	_____	_____
_____	_____	_____	_____
_____	_____	_____	_____
_____	_____	_____	_____
_____	_____	_____	_____
L_____	_____	S_____	_____
_____	_____	_____	_____
_____	_____	_____	_____
_____	_____	_____	_____
_____	_____	TOTAL CALORIES/POINTS _____	

DATE ___ / ___ / ___ TO ___ / ___ / ___

FOODS	CALORIES/ POINTS	FOODS	CALORIES/ POINTS
B_____ ____		D_____ ____	
_____ ____		_____ ____	
_____ ____		_____ ____	
_____ ____		_____ ____	
_____ ____		_____ ____	
_____ ____		_____ ____	
L_____ ____		S_____ ____	
_____ ____		_____ ____	
_____ ____		_____ ____	
_____ ____		_____ ____	
_____ ____			
_____ ____		TOTAL CALORIES/POINTS ____	

FOODS	CALORIES/ POINTS	FOODS	CALORIES/ POINTS
B_____ ____		D_____ ____	
_____ ____		_____ ____	
_____ ____		_____ ____	
_____ ____		_____ ____	
_____ ____		_____ ____	
_____ ____		_____ ____	
L_____ ____		S_____ ____	
_____ ____		_____ ____	
_____ ____		_____ ____	
_____ ____		_____ ____	
_____ ____			
_____ ____		TOTAL CALORIES/POINTS ____	

Calories/Points Tracker

DAILY GOAL

FRI

FOODS	CALORIES/POINTS	FOODS	CALORIES/POINTS
B_____	____	D_____	____
_____	____	_____	____
_____	____	_____	____
_____	____	_____	____
_____	____	_____	____
_____	____	_____	____
L_____	____	S_____	____
_____	____	_____	____
_____	____	_____	____
_____	____	_____	____
_____	____	_____	____
_____	____	TOTAL CALORIES/POINTS ____	

SAT

FOODS	CALORIES/POINTS	FOODS	CALORIES/POINTS
B_____	____	D_____	____
_____	____	_____	____
_____	____	_____	____
_____	____	_____	____
_____	____	_____	____
L_____	____	_____	____
_____	____	S_____	____
_____	____	_____	____
_____	____	_____	____
_____	____	_____	____
_____	____	TOTAL CALORIES/POINTS ____	

DATE ___/___/___ TO ___/___/___

FOODS	CALORIES/POINTS	FOODS	CALORIES/POINTS
B_____	_____	D_____	_____
_____	_____	_____	_____
_____	_____	_____	_____
_____	_____	_____	_____
_____	_____	_____	_____
_____	_____	_____	_____
L_____	_____	S_____	_____
_____	_____	_____	_____
_____	_____	_____	_____
_____	_____	_____	_____
_____	_____		
_____	_____	TOTAL CALORIES/POINTS _____

––––––––– Exercise Tracker –––––––––

ACTIVITY	DISTANCE/DURATION/INTENSITY	CALORIES BURNED
_____	_____	_____
_____	_____	_____
_____	_____	_____
_____	_____	_____
_____	_____	_____
_____	_____	_____
_____	_____	_____
_____	_____	_____

Garlic Lover's Roast Beef

SERVES 10

2½ pounds top round roast,
     fat trimmed

3 to 4 garlic cloves, cut into thin
   slivers

   Olive oil spray (I use my Misto)

2 teaspoons dried rosemary,
   chopped

2 teaspoons kosher salt

   Freshly ground black pepper

SERVING SIZE	3 ounces beef
CALORIES	143
FAT	4 g
CHOLESTEROL	44 mg
CARBOHYDRATE	0.5 g
FIBER	0 g
PROTEIN	24 g
SUGAR	0 g
SODIUM	292 mg

Remove the roast from the refrigerator 1 hour before cooking to allow it to reach room temperature.

Preheat the oven to 350°F.

Using a sharp knife, pierce the meat all over about ½-inch deep and insert slivers of garlic into each hole, pushing all the way in. Lightly spray the meat with olive oil, sprinkle with the rosemary and salt, and season generously with pepper. Place a meat thermometer all the way into the center of the meat, and put the roast in a roasting pan.

Roast in the oven until the thermometer reads 130°F for rare, 140°F for medium rare, 150°F for medium, and 155-160°F for well done. (Note that the temperature will rise an additional 5 degrees as it sits.) Remove the roast from the oven and let rest for 10 to 20 minutes before carving.

Thinly slice the meat and serve.

Weekly Meal Planner

Weekly Goals _____

_____

_____

_____

_____

> "If you ask me what
> I came into this life
> to do, I will tell you:
> I came to live out
> loud."
>
> — ÉMILE ZOLA

MON

_____
_____
_____
_____

TUE

_____
_____
_____
_____

WED

_____
_____
_____
_____

THU

FRI

SAT

SUN

Calories/Points Tracker

DAILY GOAL

MON

FOODS | **CALORIES/POINTS**

B _____ _____
_____ _____
_____ _____
_____ _____
_____ _____
_____ _____

L _____ _____
_____ _____
_____ _____
_____ _____
_____ _____

FOODS | **CALORIES/POINTS**

D _____ _____
_____ _____
_____ _____
_____ _____
_____ _____
_____ _____

S _____ _____
_____ _____
_____ _____
_____ _____

TOTAL CALORIES/POINTS _____

TUE

FOODS | **CALORIES/POINTS**

B _____ _____
_____ _____
_____ _____
_____ _____
_____ _____
_____ _____

L _____ _____
_____ _____
_____ _____
_____ _____
_____ _____

FOODS | **CALORIES/POINTS**

D _____ _____
_____ _____
_____ _____
_____ _____
_____ _____
_____ _____

S _____ _____
_____ _____
_____ _____
_____ _____

TOTAL CALORIES/POINTS _____

DATE ____ / ____ / ____ TO ____ / ____ / ____

FOODS	CALORIES/POINTS	FOODS	CALORIES/POINTS

WED

B _____ _____

_____ _____

_____ _____

_____ _____

_____ _____

_____ _____

L _____ _____

_____ _____

_____ _____

_____ _____

_____ _____

_____ _____

D _____ _____

_____ _____

_____ _____

_____ _____

_____ _____

_____ _____

S _____ _____

_____ _____

_____ _____

_____ _____

TOTAL CALORIES/POINTS _____

THU

FOODS	CALORIES/POINTS	FOODS	CALORIES/POINTS

B _____ _____

_____ _____

_____ _____

_____ _____

_____ _____

_____ _____

L _____ _____

_____ _____

_____ _____

_____ _____

_____ _____

_____ _____

D _____ _____

_____ _____

_____ _____

_____ _____

_____ _____

_____ _____

S _____ _____

_____ _____

_____ _____

_____ _____

TOTAL CALORIES/POINTS _____

Calories/Points Tracker

DAILY GOAL _____

FRI

FOODS	CALORIES/POINTS	FOODS	CALORIES/POINTS
B_____	_____	D_____	_____
_____	_____	_____	_____
_____	_____	_____	_____
_____	_____	_____	_____
_____	_____	_____	_____
_____	_____	_____	_____
L_____	_____	S_____	_____
_____	_____	_____	_____
_____	_____	_____	_____
_____	_____	_____	_____
_____	_____		
_____	_____	TOTAL CALORIES/POINTS _____	

SAT

FOODS	CALORIES/POINTS	FOODS	CALORIES/POINTS
B_____	_____	D_____	_____
_____	_____	_____	_____
_____	_____	_____	_____
_____	_____	_____	_____
_____	_____	_____	_____
_____	_____	_____	_____
L_____	_____	S_____	_____
_____	_____	_____	_____
_____	_____	_____	_____
_____	_____	_____	_____
_____	_____		
_____	_____	TOTAL CALORIES/POINTS _____	

DATE _____ / _____ / _____ TO _____ / _____ / _____

FOODS	CALORIES/ POINTS	FOODS	CALORIES/ POINTS
B_____ _____		D_____ _____	
_____ _____		_____ _____	
_____ _____		_____ _____	
_____ _____		_____ _____	
_____ _____		_____ _____	
_____ _____		_____ _____	
L_____ _____		S_____ _____	
_____ _____		_____ _____	
_____ _____		_____ _____	
_____ _____		_____ _____	
_____ _____			
_____ _____		TOTAL CALORIES/POINTS _____	

Exercise Tracker

ACTIVITY	DISTANCE/ DURATION/INTENSITY	CALORIES BURNED
_____	_____	_____
_____	_____	_____
_____	_____	_____
_____	_____	_____
_____	_____	_____
_____	_____	_____
_____	_____	_____
_____	_____	_____

Weekly Meal Planner

Weekly Goals _____

_____

_____

_____

_____

"Be in love with
your life. Every
minute of it."

JACK KEROUAC

MON

TUE

WED

Calories/Points Tracker

DAILY GOAL

MON

FOODS	CALORIES/POINTS
B_____	_____
_____	_____
_____	_____
_____	_____
_____	_____
_____	_____
L_____	_____
_____	_____
_____	_____
_____	_____
_____	_____
_____	_____

FOODS	CALORIES/POINTS
D_____	_____
_____	_____
_____	_____
_____	_____
_____	_____
_____	_____
S_____	_____
_____	_____
_____	_____
_____	_____
TOTAL CALORIES/POINTS	_____

TUE

FOODS	CALORIES/POINTS
B_____	_____
_____	_____
_____	_____
_____	_____
_____	_____
_____	_____
L_____	_____
_____	_____
_____	_____
_____	_____
_____	_____
_____	_____

FOODS	CALORIES/POINTS
D_____	_____
_____	_____
_____	_____
_____	_____
_____	_____
_____	_____
S_____	_____
_____	_____
_____	_____
_____	_____
TOTAL CALORIES/POINTS	_____

DATE ___ / ___ / ___ TO ___ / ___ / ___

FOODS	CALORIES/ POINTS	FOODS	CALORIES/ POINTS
B _____	_____	D _____	_____
_____	_____	_____	_____
_____	_____	_____	_____
_____	_____	_____	_____
_____	_____	_____	_____
_____	_____	_____	_____
L _____	_____	S _____	_____
_____	_____	_____	_____
_____	_____	_____	_____
_____	_____	_____	_____
_____	_____	_____	_____
_____	_____	TOTAL CALORIES/POINTS _____

FOODS	CALORIES/ POINTS	FOODS	CALORIES/ POINTS
B _____	_____	D _____	_____
_____	_____	_____	_____
_____	_____	_____	_____
_____	_____	_____	_____
_____	_____	_____	_____
_____	_____	_____	_____
L _____	_____	S _____	_____
_____	_____	_____	_____
_____	_____	_____	_____
_____	_____	_____	_____
_____	_____	_____	_____
_____	_____	TOTAL CALORIES/POINTS _____

Calories/Points Tracker

DAILY GOAL _____

FRI

FOODS	CALORIES/POINTS		FOODS	CALORIES/POINTS
B _____	_____		D _____	_____
_____	_____		_____	_____
_____	_____		_____	_____
_____	_____		_____	_____
_____	_____		_____	_____
_____	_____		_____	_____
L _____	_____		S _____	_____
_____	_____		_____	_____
_____	_____		_____	_____
_____	_____		_____	_____
_____	_____			
_____	_____		TOTAL CALORIES/POINTS	_____

SAT

FOODS	CALORIES/POINTS		FOODS	CALORIES/POINTS
B _____	_____		D _____	_____
_____	_____		_____	_____
_____	_____		_____	_____
_____	_____		_____	_____
_____	_____		_____	_____
_____	_____		_____	_____
L _____	_____		S _____	_____
_____	_____		_____	_____
_____	_____		_____	_____
_____	_____		_____	_____
_____	_____			
_____	_____		TOTAL CALORIES/POINTS	_____

DATE ____/____/____ TO ____/____/____

FOODS	CALORIES/ POINTS	FOODS	CALORIES/ POINTS
B_____	_____	D_____	_____
_____	_____	_____	_____
_____	_____	_____	_____
_____	_____	_____	_____
_____	_____	_____	_____
_____	_____		
L_____	_____	S_____	_____
_____	_____	_____	_____
_____	_____	_____	_____
_____	_____	_____	_____
_____	_____		
_____	_____	TOTAL CALORIES/POINTS _____	

—————— Exercise Tracker ——————

ACTIVITY	DISTANCE/ DURATION/INTENSITY	CALORIES BURNED
_____	_____	_____
_____	_____	_____
_____	_____	_____
_____	_____	_____
_____	_____	_____
_____	_____	_____
_____	_____	_____

Weekly Meal Planner

Weekly Goals _____

_____

_____

_____

_____

superfood

OLIVE OIL

This healthy oil should always be at hand in your kitchen! Use it wherever possible in place of other oils or butter.

MON

_____
_____
_____
_____

TUE

_____
_____
_____
_____

WED

_____
_____
_____
_____

THU

FRI

SAT

SUN

Calories/Points Tracker

DAILY GOAL

MON

FOODS | CALORIES/POINTS

B _____ _____
_____ _____
_____ _____
_____ _____
_____ _____
_____ _____

L _____ _____
_____ _____
_____ _____
_____ _____
_____ _____
_____ _____

FOODS | CALORIES/POINTS

D _____ _____
_____ _____
_____ _____
_____ _____
_____ _____

S _____ _____
_____ _____
_____ _____
_____ _____

TOTAL CALORIES/POINTS _____

TUE

FOODS | CALORIES/POINTS

B _____ _____
_____ _____
_____ _____
_____ _____
_____ _____
_____ _____

L _____ _____
_____ _____
_____ _____
_____ _____
_____ _____
_____ _____

FOODS | CALORIES/POINTS

D _____ _____
_____ _____
_____ _____
_____ _____
_____ _____

S _____ _____
_____ _____
_____ _____
_____ _____

TOTAL CALORIES/POINTS _____

DATE _____ / _____ / _____ TO _____ / _____ / _____

FOODS	CALORIES/ POINTS	FOODS	CALORIES/ POINTS
B _____	_____	D _____	_____
_____	_____	_____	_____
_____	_____	_____	_____
_____	_____	_____	_____
_____	_____	_____	_____
_____	_____	_____	_____
L _____	_____	S _____	_____
_____	_____	_____	_____
_____	_____	_____	_____
_____	_____	_____	_____
_____	_____		
_____	_____	TOTAL CALORIES/POINTS _____	

FOODS	CALORIES/ POINTS	FOODS	CALORIES/ POINTS
B _____	_____	D _____	_____
_____	_____	_____	_____
_____	_____	_____	_____
_____	_____	_____	_____
_____	_____	_____	_____
_____	_____	_____	_____
L _____	_____	S _____	_____
_____	_____	_____	_____
_____	_____	_____	_____
_____	_____	_____	_____
_____	_____		
_____	_____	TOTAL CALORIES/POINTS _____	

Calories/Points Tracker

DAILY GOAL

FRI

FOODS	CALORIES/POINTS	FOODS	CALORIES/POINTS
B _____	____	D _____	____
_____	____	_____	____
_____	____	_____	____
_____	____	_____	____
_____	____	_____	____
_____	____	_____	____
L _____	____	S _____	____
_____	____	_____	____
_____	____	_____	____
_____	____	_____	____
_____	____	_____	____
_____	____	TOTAL CALORIES/POINTS ____	

SAT

FOODS	CALORIES/POINTS	FOODS	CALORIES/POINTS
B _____	____	D _____	____
_____	____	_____	____
_____	____	_____	____
_____	____	_____	____
_____	____	_____	____
_____	____	_____	____
L _____	____	S _____	____
_____	____	_____	____
_____	____	_____	____
_____	____	_____	____
_____	____	_____	____
_____	____	TOTAL CALORIES/POINTS ____	

SUN

DATE ___ / ___ / ___ TO ___ / ___ / ___

FOODS	CALORIES/ POINTS	FOODS	CALORIES/ POINTS
B_____	_____	D_____	_____
_____	_____	_____	_____
_____	_____	_____	_____
_____	_____	_____	_____
_____	_____	_____	_____
_____	_____	_____	_____
L_____	_____	S_____	_____
_____	_____	_____	_____
_____	_____	_____	_____
_____	_____	_____	_____
_____	_____		
_____	_____	TOTAL CALORIES/POINTS _____	

─────────── Exercise Tracker ───────────

ACTIVITY	DISTANCE/ DURATION/INTENSITY	CALORIES BURNED
_____	_____	_____
_____	_____	_____
_____	_____	_____
_____	_____	_____
_____	_____	_____
_____	_____	_____
_____	_____	_____

String Beans with Garlic and Oil

SERVES 4

- **1 pound fresh string beans, ends trimmed**
- **2 tablespoons extra-virgin olive oil**
- **4 garlic cloves, thinly sliced**
- **¼ teaspoon kosher salt**
- **Freshly ground black pepper**

SERVING SIZE	1 cup
CALORIES	99
FAT	7 g
CHOLESTEROL	0 mg
CARBOHYDRATE	9 g
FIBER	4 g
PROTEIN	2 g
SUGAR	0 g
SODIUM	77 mg

Bring a large saucepan filled with 1 inch of water to a boil. Lower a steamer basket filled with the green beans into it, tightly cover the pan, and steam until the beans are crisp tender, 4 to 5 minutes. Drain.

In a sauté pan set over medium-high heat, heat the olive oil. When hot add the garlic and cook until golden, about 30 seconds. Add the beans and salt, season with pepper, and toss well. Serve.

Quinoa, Chickpea, and Avocado Salad

MAKES 5 CUPS; SERVES 4

1 cup quartered grape tomatoes

1 (15-ounce) can garbanzo beans, rinsed and drained

1 cup cooked quinoa

2 tablespoons finely chopped red onion

2 tablespoons finely chopped cilantro

Juice of 1½ limes

½ plus ⅛ teaspoon kosher salt

Freshly ground black pepper

1 cup chopped cucumber

1 small Hass avocado, chopped (4 ounces)

In a medium bowl, combine the tomatoes, garbanzo beans, quinoa, onion, cilantro, lime juice, and ½ teaspoon of the salt, and season with pepper. Keep refrigerated until ready to serve.

Just before serving, toss in the cucumber and avocado and season with the remaining ⅛ teaspoon salt.

SERVING SIZE	1¼ cups
CALORIES	248
FAT	7 g
CHOLESTEROL	0 mg
CARBOHYDRATE	41 g
FIBER	8 g
PROTEIN	8.5 g
SUGAR	1 g
SODIUM	578 mg

Weekly Meal Planner

Weekly Goals _____

_____

_____

_____

_____

MON

TUE

WED

Calories/Points Tracker

DAILY GOAL

FOODS	CALORIES/ POINTS
B _____	_____
_____	_____
_____	_____
_____	_____
_____	_____
_____	_____
L _____	_____
_____	_____
_____	_____
_____	_____
_____	_____
_____	_____

FOODS	CALORIES/ POINTS
D _____	_____
_____	_____
_____	_____
_____	_____
_____	_____
_____	_____
S _____	_____
_____	_____
_____	_____
_____	_____

TOTAL CALORIES/POINTS _____

MON

FOODS	CALORIES/ POINTS
B _____	_____
_____	_____
_____	_____
_____	_____
_____	_____
_____	_____
L _____	_____
_____	_____
_____	_____
_____	_____
_____	_____
_____	_____

FOODS	CALORIES/ POINTS
D _____	_____
_____	_____
_____	_____
_____	_____
_____	_____
_____	_____
S _____	_____
_____	_____
_____	_____
_____	_____

TOTAL CALORIES/POINTS _____

TUE

FOODS	CALORIES/ POINTS	FOODS	CALORIES/ POINTS
B _____	_____	D _____	_____
_____	_____	_____	_____
_____	_____	_____	_____
_____	_____	_____	_____
_____	_____	_____	_____
_____	_____	_____	_____
L _____	_____	S _____	_____
_____	_____	_____	_____
_____	_____	_____	_____
_____	_____	_____	_____
_____	_____		
_____	_____	TOTAL CALORIES/POINTS _____	

FOODS	CALORIES/ POINTS	FOODS	CALORIES/ POINTS
B _____	_____	D _____	_____
_____	_____	_____	_____
_____	_____	_____	_____
_____	_____	_____	_____
_____	_____	_____	_____
_____	_____	_____	_____
L _____	_____	S _____	_____
_____	_____	_____	_____
_____	_____	_____	_____
_____	_____	_____	_____
_____	_____		
_____	_____	TOTAL CALORIES/POINTS _____	

Calories/Points Tracker

DAILY GOAL

FRI

FOODS	CALORIES/POINTS
B_____	_____
_____	_____
_____	_____
_____	_____
_____	_____
_____	_____
L_____	_____
_____	_____
_____	_____
_____	_____
_____	_____
_____	_____

FOODS	CALORIES/POINTS
D_____	_____
_____	_____
_____	_____
_____	_____
_____	_____
S_____	_____
_____	_____
_____	_____
_____	_____

TOTAL CALORIES/POINTS _____

SAT

FOODS	CALORIES/POINTS
B_____	_____
_____	_____
_____	_____
_____	_____
_____	_____
_____	_____
L_____	_____
_____	_____
_____	_____
_____	_____
_____	_____
_____	_____

FOODS	CALORIES/POINTS
D_____	_____
_____	_____
_____	_____
_____	_____
_____	_____
S_____	_____
_____	_____
_____	_____
_____	_____

TOTAL CALORIES/POINTS _____

DATE ___ / ___ / ___ TO ___ / ___ / ___

FOODS	CALORIES/ POINTS	FOODS	CALORIES/ POINTS
B _____	___	D _____	___
_____	___	_____	___
_____	___	_____	___
_____	___	_____	___
_____	___	_____	___
_____	___	_____	___
L _____	___	S _____	___
_____	___	_____	___
_____	___	_____	___
_____	___	_____	___
_____	___		
_____	___	TOTAL CALORIES/POINTS ___	

———————————— Exercise Tracker ————————————

ACTIVITY	DISTANCE/ DURATION/INTENSITY	CALORIES BURNED
_____	_____	_____
_____	_____	_____
_____	_____	_____
_____	_____	_____
_____	_____	_____
_____	_____	_____
_____	_____	_____
_____	_____	_____

Weekly Meal Planner

Weekly Goals _____

_____

_____

_____

_____

superfood

AVOCADOS

With a subtle flavor and creamy texture, avocados are really versatile. Try avocado toast: toasted bread topped with mashed avocado and sea salt.

MON

TUE

WED

DATE ___ / ___ / ___ TO ___ / ___ / ___

THU

FRI

SAT

SUN

Calories/Points Tracker

DAILY GOAL _____

MON

FOODS	CALORIES/ POINTS		FOODS	CALORIES/ POINTS
B_____	_____		D_____	_____
_____	_____		_____	_____
_____	_____		_____	_____
_____	_____		_____	_____
_____	_____		_____	_____
_____	_____		_____	_____
L_____	_____		S_____	_____
_____	_____		_____	_____
_____	_____		_____	_____
_____	_____		_____	_____
_____	_____			
_____	_____		TOTAL CALORIES/POINTS _____	

TUE

FOODS	CALORIES/ POINTS		FOODS	CALORIES/ POINTS
B_____	_____		D_____	_____
_____	_____		_____	_____
_____	_____		_____	_____
_____	_____		_____	_____
_____	_____		_____	_____
_____	_____		_____	_____
L_____	_____		S_____	_____
_____	_____		_____	_____
_____	_____		_____	_____
_____	_____		_____	_____
_____	_____			
_____	_____		TOTAL CALORIES/POINTS _____	

DATE ____ / ____ / ____ TO ____ / ____ / ____

FOODS	CALORIES/ POINTS	FOODS	CALORIES/ POINTS
B _____	_____	D _____	_____
_____	_____	_____	_____
_____	_____	_____	_____
_____	_____	_____	_____
_____	_____	_____	_____
_____	_____	_____	_____
L _____	_____	S _____	_____
_____	_____	_____	_____
_____	_____	_____	_____
_____	_____	_____	_____
_____	_____		
_____	_____	TOTAL CALORIES/POINTS _____	

FOODS	CALORIES/ POINTS	FOODS	CALORIES/ POINTS
B _____	_____	D _____	_____
_____	_____	_____	_____
_____	_____	_____	_____
_____	_____	_____	_____
_____	_____	_____	_____
_____	_____	_____	_____
L _____	_____	S _____	_____
_____	_____	_____	_____
_____	_____	_____	_____
_____	_____	_____	_____
_____	_____		
_____	_____	TOTAL CALORIES/POINTS _____	

Calories/Points Tracker

DAILY GOAL _____

FRI

FOODS   CALORIES/POINTS

B _____ _____
_____ _____
_____ _____
_____ _____
_____ _____
_____ _____

L _____ _____
_____ _____
_____ _____
_____ _____
_____ _____
_____ _____

FOODS   CALORIES/POINTS

D _____ _____
_____ _____
_____ _____
_____ _____
_____ _____

S _____ _____
_____ _____
_____ _____
_____ _____

TOTAL CALORIES/POINTS _____

SAT

FOODS   CALORIES/POINTS

B _____ _____
_____ _____
_____ _____
_____ _____
_____ _____

L _____ _____
_____ _____
_____ _____
_____ _____
_____ _____

FOODS   CALORIES/POINTS

D _____ _____
_____ _____
_____ _____
_____ _____
_____ _____
_____ _____

S _____ _____
_____ _____
_____ _____
_____ _____

TOTAL CALORIES/POINTS _____

DATE ____ / ____ / ____ TO ____ / ____ / ____

FOODS	CALORIES/ POINTS	FOODS	CALORIES/ POINTS
B_____	_____	D_____	_____
_____	_____	_____	_____
_____	_____	_____	_____
_____	_____	_____	_____
_____	_____	_____	_____
_____	_____	_____	_____
L_____	_____	S_____	_____
_____	_____	_____	_____
_____	_____	_____	_____
_____	_____	_____	_____
_____	_____	TOTAL CALORIES/POINTS _____
_____	_____		

--- Exercise Tracker ---

ACTIVITY	DISTANCE/ DURATION/INTENSITY	CALORIES BURNED
_____	_____	_____
_____	_____	_____
_____	_____	_____
_____	_____	_____
_____	_____	_____
_____	_____	_____
_____	_____	_____
_____	_____	_____

Weekly Meal Planner

Weekly Goals _____

_____

_____

_____

_____

> "Once you choose hope, anything's possible."
>
> CHRISTOPHER REEVE

MON

TUE

WED

THU

FRI

SAT

SUN

Calories/Points Tracker

DAILY GOAL _____

MON

FOODS	CALORIES/POINTS	FOODS	CALORIES/POINTS
B _____	_____	D _____	_____
_____	_____	_____	_____
_____	_____	_____	_____
_____	_____	_____	_____
_____	_____	_____	_____
_____	_____	_____	_____
L _____	_____	S _____	_____
_____	_____	_____	_____
_____	_____	_____	_____
_____	_____	_____	_____
_____	_____		
_____	_____	TOTAL CALORIES/POINTS _____	

TUE

FOODS	CALORIES/POINTS	FOODS	CALORIES/POINTS
B _____	_____	D _____	_____
_____	_____	_____	_____
_____	_____	_____	_____
_____	_____	_____	_____
_____	_____	_____	_____
_____	_____	_____	_____
L _____	_____	S _____	_____
_____	_____	_____	_____
_____	_____	_____	_____
_____	_____	_____	_____
_____	_____		
_____	_____	TOTAL CALORIES/POINTS _____	

WED
THU

DATE ____ / ____ / ____ TO ____ / ____ / ____

FOODS	CALORIES/ POINTS	FOODS	CALORIES/ POINTS
B _____	____	D _____	____
_____	____	_____	____
_____	____	_____	____
_____	____	_____	____
_____	____	_____	____
_____	____	_____	____
L _____	____	S _____	____
_____	____	_____	____
_____	____	_____	____
_____	____	_____	____
_____	____	TOTAL CALORIES/POINTS ____	
_____	____		

FOODS	CALORIES/ POINTS	FOODS	CALORIES/ POINTS
B _____	____	D _____	____
_____	____	_____	____
_____	____	_____	____
_____	____	_____	____
_____	____	_____	____
_____	____	_____	____
L _____	____	S _____	____
_____	____	_____	____
_____	____	_____	____
_____	____	_____	____
_____	____	TOTAL CALORIES/POINTS ____	
_____	____		

Calories/Points Tracker

DAILY GOAL

FOODS	CALORIES/ POINTS	FOODS	CALORIES/ POINTS
B _____	_____	D _____	_____
_____	_____	_____	_____
_____	_____	_____	_____
_____	_____	_____	_____
_____	_____	_____	_____
_____	_____	_____	_____
L _____	_____	S _____	_____
_____	_____	_____	_____
_____	_____	_____	_____
_____	_____	_____	_____
_____	_____	_____	_____
_____	_____	TOTAL CALORIES/POINTS _____

FRI

FOODS	CALORIES/ POINTS	FOODS	CALORIES/ POINTS
B _____	_____	D _____	_____
_____	_____	_____	_____
_____	_____	_____	_____
_____	_____	_____	_____
_____	_____	_____	_____
_____	_____	_____	_____
L _____	_____	S _____	_____
_____	_____	_____	_____
_____	_____	_____	_____
_____	_____	_____	_____
_____	_____	_____	_____
_____	_____	TOTAL CALORIES/POINTS _____

SAT

DATE ___/___/___ TO ___/___/___

FOODS	CALORIES/POINTS	FOODS	CALORIES/POINTS
B_____	___	D_____	___
_____	___	_____	___
_____	___	_____	___
_____	___	_____	___
_____	___	_____	___
_____	___	_____	___
L_____	___	S_____	___
_____	___	_____	___
_____	___	_____	___
_____	___	_____	___
_____	___		
_____	___	TOTAL CALORIES/POINTS ___	

—————— Exercise Tracker ——————

ACTIVITY	DISTANCE/DURATION/INTENSITY	CALORIES BURNED
_____	_____	_____
_____	_____	_____
_____	_____	_____
_____	_____	_____
_____	_____	_____
_____	_____	_____
_____	_____	_____

Weekly Meal Planner

Weekly Goals _____

_____

_____

_____

_____

"Every moment
is a fresh
beginning."

T. S. ELIOT

MON

TUE

WED

THU

FRI

SAT

SUN

Calories/Points Tracker

DAILY GOAL _____

MON

FOODS	CALORIES/POINTS	FOODS	CALORIES/POINTS
B _____	___	D _____	___
_____	___	_____	___
_____	___	_____	___
_____	___	_____	___
_____	___	_____	___
_____	___	_____	___
L _____	___	S _____	___
_____	___	_____	___
_____	___	_____	___
_____	___	_____	___
_____	___	TOTAL CALORIES/POINTS ___	

TUE

FOODS	CALORIES/POINTS	FOODS	CALORIES/POINTS
B _____	___	D _____	___
_____	___	_____	___
_____	___	_____	___
_____	___	_____	___
_____	___	_____	___
_____	___	_____	___
L _____	___	S _____	___
_____	___	_____	___
_____	___	_____	___
_____	___	_____	___
_____	___	TOTAL CALORIES/POINTS ___	

WED

FOODS	CALORIES/POINTS	FOODS	CALORIES/POINTS
B _____	_____	D _____	_____
_____	_____	_____	_____
_____	_____	_____	_____
_____	_____	_____	_____
_____	_____	_____	_____
_____	_____	_____	_____
L _____	_____	S _____	_____
_____	_____	_____	_____
_____	_____	_____	_____
_____	_____	_____	_____
_____	_____		
_____	_____	TOTAL CALORIES/POINTS _____	

THU

FOODS	CALORIES/POINTS	FOODS	CALORIES/POINTS
B _____	_____	D _____	_____
_____	_____	_____	_____
_____	_____	_____	_____
_____	_____	_____	_____
_____	_____	_____	_____
_____	_____	_____	_____
L _____	_____	S _____	_____
_____	_____	_____	_____
_____	_____	_____	_____
_____	_____	_____	_____
_____	_____		
_____	_____	TOTAL CALORIES/POINTS _____	

Calories/Points Tracker

FRI

FOODS	CALORIES/ POINTS	FOODS	CALORIES/ POINTS
B_____	_____	D_____	_____
_____	_____	_____	_____
_____	_____	_____	_____
_____	_____	_____	_____
_____	_____	_____	_____
_____	_____	_____	_____
L_____	_____	S_____	_____
_____	_____	_____	_____
_____	_____	_____	_____
_____	_____	_____	_____
_____	_____		
_____	_____	TOTAL CALORIES/POINTS _____	

SAT

FOODS	CALORIES/ POINTS	FOODS	CALORIES/ POINTS
B_____	_____	D_____	_____
_____	_____	_____	_____
_____	_____	_____	_____
_____	_____	_____	_____
_____	_____	_____	_____
_____	_____	_____	_____
L_____	_____	S_____	_____
_____	_____	_____	_____
_____	_____	_____	_____
_____	_____	_____	_____
_____	_____		
_____	_____	TOTAL CALORIES/POINTS _____	

DATE ___ / ___ / ___ TO ___ / ___ / ___

FOODS	CALORIES/POINTS	FOODS	CALORIES/POINTS
B_____	____	D_____	____
_____	____	_____	____
_____	____	_____	____
_____	____	_____	____
_____	____	_____	____
_____	____	_____	____
L_____	____	S_____	____
_____	____	_____	____
_____	____	_____	____
_____	____	_____	____
_____	____	TOTAL CALORIES/POINTS ____

—————— Exercise Tracker ——————

ACTIVITY	DISTANCE/DURATION/INTENSITY	CALORIES BURNED
_____	_____	_____
_____	_____	_____
_____	_____	_____
_____	_____	_____
_____	_____	_____
_____	_____	_____
_____	_____	_____

Weekly Meal Planner

Weekly Goals _____

_____

_____

_____

_____

superfood

TOMATOES

Take advantage of those gorgeous summer tomatoes! Slice heirloom varieties for a stunning salad, and make a weekend project out of canning fresh sauce. You'll be thankful come winter!

MON

_____
_____
_____
_____

TUE

_____
_____
_____
_____

WED

_____
_____
_____
_____

Calories/Points Tracker

MON

FOODS	CALORIES/POINTS	FOODS	CALORIES/POINTS
B		D	
L		S	
		TOTAL CALORIES/POINTS	

TUE

FOODS	CALORIES/POINTS	FOODS	CALORIES/POINTS
B		D	
L		S	
		TOTAL CALORIES/POINTS	

DATE ____ / ____ / ____ TO ____ / ____ / ____

FOODS	CALORIES/ POINTS	FOODS	CALORIES/ POINTS
B _____ ____		D _____ ____	
_____ ____		_____ ____	
_____ ____		_____ ____	
_____ ____		_____ ____	
_____ ____		_____ ____	
_____ ____		_____ ____	
L _____ ____		S _____ ____	
_____ ____		_____ ____	
_____ ____		_____ ____	
_____ ____		_____ ____	
_____ ____		TOTAL CALORIES/POINTS ____	

FOODS	CALORIES/ POINTS	FOODS	CALORIES/ POINTS
B _____ ____		D _____ ____	
_____ ____		_____ ____	
_____ ____		_____ ____	
_____ ____		_____ ____	
_____ ____		_____ ____	
_____ ____		_____ ____	
L _____ ____		S _____ ____	
_____ ____		_____ ____	
_____ ____		_____ ____	
_____ ____		_____ ____	
_____ ____		TOTAL CALORIES/POINTS ____	

Calories/Points Tracker

DAILY GOAL _____

FRI

FOODS	CALORIES/POINTS	FOODS	CALORIES/POINTS
B _____	_____	D _____	_____
_____	_____	_____	_____
_____	_____	_____	_____
_____	_____	_____	_____
_____	_____	_____	_____
L _____	_____	S _____	_____
_____	_____	_____	_____
_____	_____	_____	_____
_____	_____	_____	_____
_____	_____		
_____	_____	TOTAL CALORIES/POINTS _____

SAT

FOODS	CALORIES/POINTS	FOODS	CALORIES/POINTS
B _____	_____	D _____	_____
_____	_____	_____	_____
_____	_____	_____	_____
_____	_____	_____	_____
_____	_____	_____	_____
L _____	_____	S _____	_____
_____	_____	_____	_____
_____	_____	_____	_____
_____	_____	_____	_____
_____	_____		
_____	_____	TOTAL CALORIES/POINTS _____

DATE ___/___/___ TO ___/___/___

FOODS	CALORIES/POINTS	FOODS	CALORIES/POINTS
B_____	____	D_____	____
_____	____	_____	____
_____	____	_____	____
_____	____	_____	____
_____	____	_____	____
_____	____	_____	____
L_____	____	S_____	____
_____	____	_____	____
_____	____	_____	____
_____	____	_____	____
_____	____		
_____	____	TOTAL CALORIES/POINTS ____	

——————— Exercise Tracker ———————

ACTIVITY	DISTANCE/DURATION/INTENSITY	CALORIES BURNED
_____	_____	_____
_____	_____	_____
_____	_____	_____
_____	_____	_____
_____	_____	_____
_____	_____	_____
_____	_____	_____
_____	_____	_____

Weekly Meal Planner

Weekly Goals _____

_____

_____

_____

_____

MON

TUE

WED

Calories/Points Tracker

MON

FOODS	CALORIES/POINTS	FOODS	CALORIES/POINTS
B_____	_____	D_____	_____
_____	_____	_____	_____
_____	_____	_____	_____
_____	_____	_____	_____
_____	_____	_____	_____
_____	_____	_____	_____
L_____	_____	S_____	_____
_____	_____	_____	_____
_____	_____	_____	_____
_____	_____	_____	_____
_____	_____		
_____	_____	TOTAL CALORIES/POINTS _____	

TUE

FOODS	CALORIES/POINTS	FOODS	CALORIES/POINTS
B_____	_____	D_____	_____
_____	_____	_____	_____
_____	_____	_____	_____
_____	_____	_____	_____
_____	_____	_____	_____
_____	_____	_____	_____
L_____	_____	S_____	_____
_____	_____	_____	_____
_____	_____	_____	_____
_____	_____	_____	_____
_____	_____		
_____	_____	TOTAL CALORIES/POINTS _____	

WED

FOODS	CALORIES/ POINTS	FOODS	CALORIES/ POINTS
B_____	____	D_____	____
_____	____	_____	____
_____	____	_____	____
_____	____	_____	____
_____	____	_____	____
_____	____	_____	____
L_____	____	S_____	____
_____	____	_____	____
_____	____	_____	____
_____	____	_____	____
_____	____		
_____	____	TOTAL CALORIES/POINTS ____	

THU

FOODS	CALORIES/ POINTS	FOODS	CALORIES/ POINTS
B_____	____	D_____	____
_____	____	_____	____
_____	____	_____	____
_____	____	_____	____
_____	____	_____	____
L_____	____	S_____	____
_____	____	_____	____
_____	____	_____	____
_____	____	_____	____
_____	____		
_____	____	TOTAL CALORIES/POINTS ____	

Calories/Points Tracker

DAILY GOAL _____

FRI

FOODS	CALORIES/POINTS	FOODS	CALORIES/POINTS
B _____	____	D _____	____
_____	____	_____	____
_____	____	_____	____
_____	____	_____	____
_____	____	_____	____
L _____	____	S _____	____
_____	____	_____	____
_____	____	_____	____
_____	____	_____	____
_____	____	TOTAL CALORIES/POINTS ____

SAT

FOODS	CALORIES/POINTS	FOODS	CALORIES/POINTS
B _____	____	D _____	____
_____	____	_____	____
_____	____	_____	____
_____	____	_____	____
_____	____	_____	____
L _____	____	S _____	____
_____	____	_____	____
_____	____	_____	____
_____	____	_____	____
_____	____	TOTAL CALORIES/POINTS ____

SUN

DATE ____ / ____ / ____ TO ____ / ____ / ____

FOODS	CALORIES/POINTS	FOODS	CALORIES/POINTS
B_____	_____	D_____	_____
_____	_____	_____	_____
_____	_____	_____	_____
_____	_____	_____	_____
_____	_____	_____	_____
_____	_____	_____	_____
L_____	_____	S_____	_____
_____	_____	_____	_____
_____	_____	_____	_____
_____	_____	_____	_____
_____	_____		
_____	_____	TOTAL CALORIES/POINTS _____

— Exercise Tracker —

ACTIVITY	DISTANCE/DURATION/INTENSITY	CALORIES BURNED
_____	_____	_____
_____	_____	_____
_____	_____	_____
_____	_____	_____
_____	_____	_____
_____	_____	_____
_____	_____	_____

Weekly Meal Planner

Weekly Goals _____

_____

_____

_____

_____

.

> "It always seems impossible until it's done."
>
> NELSON MANDELA

MON

TUE

WED

THU

FRI

SAT

SUN

Calories/Points Tracker

DAILY GOAL _____

MON

FOODS	CALORIES/POINTS	FOODS	CALORIES/POINTS
B_____	_____	D_____	_____
_____	_____	_____	_____
_____	_____	_____	_____
_____	_____	_____	_____
_____	_____	_____	_____
_____	_____	_____	_____
L_____	_____	S_____	_____
_____	_____	_____	_____
_____	_____	_____	_____
_____	_____	_____	_____
_____	_____	_____	_____
_____	_____	TOTAL CALORIES/POINTS	_____

TUE

FOODS	CALORIES/POINTS	FOODS	CALORIES/POINTS
B_____	_____	D_____	_____
_____	_____	_____	_____
_____	_____	_____	_____
_____	_____	_____	_____
_____	_____	_____	_____
_____	_____	_____	_____
L_____	_____	S_____	_____
_____	_____	_____	_____
_____	_____	_____	_____
_____	_____	_____	_____
_____	_____	_____	_____
_____	_____	TOTAL CALORIES/POINTS	_____

WED

FOODS	CALORIES/POINTS	FOODS	CALORIES/POINTS
B_____	_____	D_____	_____
_____	_____	_____	_____
_____	_____	_____	_____
_____	_____	_____	_____
_____	_____	_____	_____
_____	_____	_____	_____
L_____	_____	S_____	_____
_____	_____	_____	_____
_____	_____	_____	_____
_____	_____	_____	_____
_____	_____	TOTAL CALORIES/POINTS _____

THU

FOODS	CALORIES/POINTS	FOODS	CALORIES/POINTS
B_____	_____	D_____	_____
_____	_____	_____	_____
_____	_____	_____	_____
_____	_____	_____	_____
_____	_____	_____	_____
_____	_____	_____	_____
L_____	_____	S_____	_____
_____	_____	_____	_____
_____	_____	_____	_____
_____	_____	_____	_____
_____	_____	TOTAL CALORIES/POINTS _____

Calories/Points Tracker

DAILY GOAL

FRI

FOODS	CALORIES/POINTS	FOODS	CALORIES/POINTS
B _____	_____	D _____	_____
_____	_____	_____	_____
_____	_____	_____	_____
_____	_____	_____	_____
_____	_____	_____	_____
_____	_____	_____	_____
L _____	_____	S _____	_____
_____	_____	_____	_____
_____	_____	_____	_____
_____	_____	_____	_____
_____	_____	_____	_____
_____	_____	TOTAL CALORIES/POINTS _____

SAT

FOODS	CALORIES/POINTS	FOODS	CALORIES/POINTS
B _____	_____	D _____	_____
_____	_____	_____	_____
_____	_____	_____	_____
_____	_____	_____	_____
_____	_____	_____	_____
_____	_____	_____	_____
L _____	_____	S _____	_____
_____	_____	_____	_____
_____	_____	_____	_____
_____	_____	_____	_____
_____	_____	_____	_____
_____	_____	TOTAL CALORIES/POINTS _____

DATE ___/___/___ TO ___/___/___

FOODS	CALORIES/POINTS	FOODS	CALORIES/POINTS
B_____	___	D_____	___
_____	___	_____	___
_____	___	_____	___
_____	___	_____	___
_____	___	_____	___
_____	___	_____	___
L_____	___	S_____	___
_____	___	_____	___
_____	___	_____	___
_____	___	_____	___
_____	___		
_____	___	TOTAL CALORIES/POINTS ___	

Exercise Tracker

ACTIVITY	DISTANCE/DURATION/INTENSITY	CALORIES BURNED
_____	_____	_____
_____	_____	_____
_____	_____	_____
_____	_____	_____
_____	_____	_____
_____	_____	_____
_____	_____	_____
_____	_____	_____

POTTER STYLE

Copyright © 2015 by Gina Homolka

Illustrations copyright © 2015 by Shutterstock

All rights reserved.

Published in the United States by Clarkson Potter/
Publishers, an imprint of the Crown Publishing Group,
a division of Penguin Random House LLC, New York.

www.crownpublishing.com
www.clarksonpotter.com

CLARKSON POTTER is a trademark and POTTER
with colophon is a registered trademark of Penguin
Random House LLC.

Skinnytaste™ is a trademark of Skinnytaste, Inc.

Library of Congress Cataloging-in-Publication Data
is available upon request.

ISBN 978-0-8041-8843-2

Printed in China

Illustrations by Shutterstock © Shizayats (carrot);
Texturis (all other vegetables and herb pattern)
Cover design by Jessie Sayward Bright
10 9 8 7 6 5 4 3 2 1

First Edition

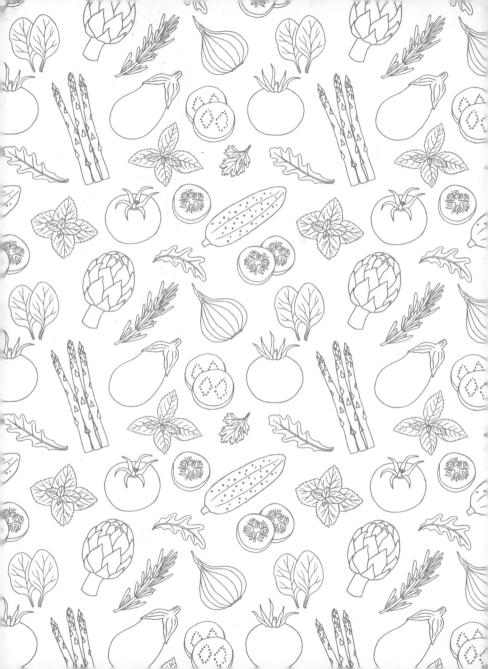